succeeding

as a

hospital
doctor

the experts share
their secrets

Roger Kirby and Tony Mundy

HEALTH PRESS

Succeeding as a Hospital Doctor
First published 2000

©2000 in this edition Health Press Limited
Health Press Limited, Elizabeth House, Queen Street, Abingdon, Oxford OX14 3JR, UK
Tel: +44 (0)1235 523233
Fax: +44 (0)1235 523238
www.healthpress.co.uk

The publisher and the authors have made every effort to ensure the accuracy of this book,
but cannot accept responsibility for any errors or omissions.

The information herein represents the independent opinions of the authors and does not
necessarily reflect the opinions and recommendations of Wyeth or the publisher.

A CIP catalogue record for this title is available from the British Library.

ISBN 1-899541-68-3

Kirby, R (Roger)
Succeeding as a Hospital Doctor/
Roger Kirby, Tony Mundy

Typeset by Zed, Oxford, UK
Printed by Fine Print (Services) Ltd, Oxford, UK

Editor's note
Although perhaps politically incorrect, it seemed to us simpler to use the pronouns
'he' and 'his' throughout rather than the more acceptable but unquestionably more
cumbersome 'he/she' and 'his/her'. We hope this will not cause offence to the very
many successful female doctors.

For Jane and Debra

Contents

Foreword

When Roger Kirby and Tony Mundy approached me to write this foreword, I thought again about what it means to be a successful doctor. My answer would be our medical professionalism. That's what makes us successful: our commitment to treat patients to the best of our ability, our enthusiasm for keeping up to date and our integrity flowing from strong professional values.

What we are witnessing today is the fashioning of a new relationship between the medical profession and the public. Since 1995, the General Medical Council (GMC) has been developing an explicit culture of professionalism in medicine that brings the public and the medical profession closer together on the qualities each expects in doctors. This in turn predicates a system of regulation in which patient safety is paramount, the language of quality improvement replaces that of misplaced professional solidarity and, in its everyday operation, responsibility for doctors' performance – and the machinery for ensuring this – is at or as close as possible to their place of work. Professionalism is the key to 21st century medicine.

Clear standards are the basis of our professionalism. The statement *Good Medical Practice*, and its core *Duties of a Doctor*, sets out the responsibilities we accept with GMC registration. Inevitably, we will not always manage to be perfect doctors, but we can all strive to be better doctors. Successful doctors understand that they, like all professionals, can sometimes fail. The ability to doubt your own practice is perhaps the strongest guarantee of continuing success in medicine. Why? Simply because it means you can recognize and understand your own weaknesses and act to put them right.

The primary responsibility for implementing, maintaining and ensuring good medical practice lies with the individual, and with the medical and clinical teams within which they work. It is the employer's responsibility to see that doctors have the time and the tools they need to make this possible. Good, quality-assured practice must be at the heart of healthcare in the NHS and the private sector, and of medical regulation. The more successful it is, the less the likelihood that things will go wrong.

Your professionalism is a precious resource in times of enormous change. Your conscience, commitment and sheer effort make a real difference to patients on a daily basis. Careers that go furthest, be it in the pursuit of greatness or in the search for rewarding work, are based on treating patients in the best possible way.

By writing this book, Roger Kirby, Tony Mundy and their colleagues have done a great service to medicine. Within it, you can find the essential ingredients for success in medicine – success that invariably depends on how much each of us remains conscientiously professional in all our dealings with patients, colleagues, students and managers.

I would like to wish all doctors who read this book well. Whatever stage you are at in your career, I hope you will find medicine as rewarding and enjoyable a career as I have.

Sir Donald Irvine
President, General Medical Council

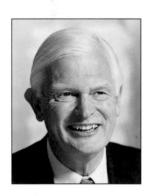

Preface

The idea for this book arose when we were asked to run a weekend course in Dublin entitled *Succeeding in Urology*. Andrew Lang and Gerard Panting were enlisted to talk about finance and medicolegal matters, respectively, and the first meeting was considered by all to be a notable success. Word spread and a waiting list soon developed for the second and subsequent meetings, which are ongoing at the time of publication.

The essence of the Dublin meeting is included here, with input from Keith Parsons on management issues, and expanded to apply equally to other less surgical disciplines. We would like to thank all of our eminent contributors who have kindly shared their own thoughts about the nature of success and how it can be achieved.

We hope that clinicians at all stages of their careers will find this book interesting, relevant and ultimately helpful. Successful doctors provide better patient care.

Roger Kirby and Tony Mundy

About the authors

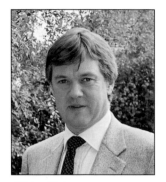

Roger Kirby

Roger Kirby trained at Cambridge and the Middlesex Hospital, and is Clinical Director of Urology at St George's Hospital, London. He also runs a busy Harley Street practice. Past Honorary Secretary of the British Association of Urological Surgeons, he launched and is Editor of *Prostate Cancer and Prostatic Diseases*. A prolific writer and speaker, he appears frequently in the media. This is his 33rd book. Roger lives with his wife and three children in Wimbledon.

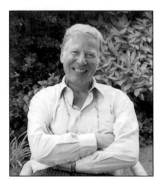

Tony Mundy

After qualifying from St Mary's Hospital Medical School, London, Tony Mundy trained in general surgery and then urology at Guy's Hospital. He is Professor of Urology at the University of London and Director of the Institute of Urology and Nephrology, which is part of University College London. He lives in the middle of nowhere in the Kent countryside with Debra and their little girl Katie.

Chapter contributors

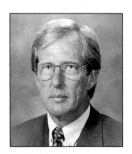

Keith Parsons
Management issues

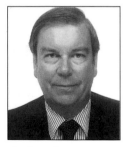

Andrew Lang
Finance

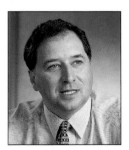

Gerard Panting
Medicolegal matters

Introduction

What is a successful hospital career? The names of many eminent doctors may spring readily to mind – indeed, several have contributed to this volume – but defining the nature and means of their success is rather more difficult. In business, a high earning capacity is considered to be the hallmark of success, and there are literally hundreds of books telling you how to achieve it. Success in medicine, however, is considerably more subtle. Perhaps the best definition of a successful doctor is one who has gained credibility from the approval and respect of patients and colleagues alike.

But how does one achieve such recognition and respect? First and foremost, be consistently ethical and professional in everything you do, remembering the words of Hippocrates, 'First do no harm'. Add to this three important principles:

- provide a high standard of practice and care
- maintain relationships of trust with patients and colleagues
- be kind, honest and trustworthy in all aspects of professional practice.

Never forget the importance of making a 'connection' with patients and colleagues. Add to this a focused training, some fruitful research, well-honed communication skills and a good position in the NHS. A consistent track record is essential, as are effective management, communication, appraisal and team-building skills. Most importantly, learn to anticipate and avoid the pitfalls that lie in wait for us all, and if you do succumb, face up to your mistakes.

So what are the benefits of success? If others perceive you as successful, this will help you as a clinician, manager and teacher. Remember, it is your reputation that goes before you and your image that is left behind – and you are only as good as your last performance. Being considered a success will make the sometimes difficult task of dealing with patients and colleagues a great deal easier. It will also help you to build a solid team as others become keen to join the bandwagon of your success.

In this book, the building blocks and formulae for success are analysed, practical ways to achieve this suggested, and advice on how to side-step the many pitfalls provided. Although this book encompasses the views of some of the UK's leading doctors, it is not intended simply for the select few who aspire to the presidency of a Royal College or chairmanship of an august medical institution. Rather, it contains something for each and every trainee, and all qualified doctors. Each of us has the potential to be a little more successful than we are. It is hoped that this book will help many doctors achieve the happiness and fulfilment that accompany a successful medical career.

Introduction

training for success: how to become a consultant

A successful career is built upon the foundation of sound training. By taking responsibility for your own training and maximizing all available opportunities, you will certainly give yourself the best chance of future success. How should you, as an individual, approach your training? What are the factors that you need to consider when applying for the consultant post of your choice?

Getting the most out of training

First, know and understand in detail what your training will involve from beginning to end. Medical training in the UK has undergone some very significant changes in recent years to bring it into line with other countries within the European Union. Second, take an active part in it. Of course, it helps to have a charming, intelligent, amusing and striking personality and to be someone who gets on well with consultants and trainees alike – but few are that lucky!

As well as acquiring practical medical and/or surgical skills during your training, you will be expected to:

- perform research (see pages 21–32)
- make presentations at meetings, initially to your own department and then at national and, perhaps, international meetings (see pages 62–7)
- acquire some management skills (see pages 101–9)
- teach medical students, nurses and doctors more junior than yourself.

The importance of research and making presentations is well established. Nowadays, since the health service reforms of the early 1990s, involvement in management is equally, if not more important for the average clinical consultant. At the very least, you should, as a trainee, aim to attend at least one management course to increase your understanding of the basics of health service management. The primary skill of management is dealing with people effectively, an attribute that will stand you in good stead at every stage of your career. Any involvement in the day-to-day management of a hospital directorate will also be to your advantage. Remember that at your consultant interview, at least two or three members of the interviewing committee will be from hospital management and will expect you to have some grasp of the management issues within the health service. It would be foolish to be unprepared.

know **what** to **expect** from **your training**

The changing nature of training

How things were

Until recently, training was by apprenticeship. It began after completion of the pre-registration house officer appointment and after full registration with the GMC had been obtained. The only fixed point in the process was appointment as a consultant in the chosen specialty. There was a ladder – through senior house officer, junior registrar and senior registrar grades – but doctors spent widely differing amounts of time at each stage and commonly moved around a great deal geographically. In doing so, they acquired experience in a large number of specialties or subspecialties before settling down in their (hopefully) preferred specialty. As a result of this usually protracted period of training, the average British consultant became extremely widely experienced and could deal competently with most medical problems. On appointment, a young consultant would be given the appropriate hospital facilities to treat his patients as he saw best. He would then acquire apprentices and facilities of his own, and the process was repeated. The hallmark of this

How to become a consultant

system was continuity of care involving a small group of doctors (houseman, registrar and omnicompetent consultant) who were able to work as an independent unit with their own facilities (ward, clinic, operating theatre and associated equipment).

Why things changed

The apprenticeship model changed for several reasons. First, the traditional specialties, and surgery in particular, became fragmented. Second, the funding crisis in the NHS, present almost since its inception, became more acute and facilities were reduced gradually as a result. Consultants were expected to share resources with colleagues. With the reduction of junior doctors' hours, continuity of care became more difficult to manage. Furthermore, increasing subspecialization required consultants to work more and more in teams. Growing managerial responsibilities and educational roles began to impinge on the clinical practice of some consultants.

At the same time, training had to be brought in line with the requirements of the European Union. A time limit needed to be set for the training period and, for the first time, an end-point for training was specified – the acquisition of a Certificate of Completion of Specialist Training (CCST). In 1996, Sir Kenneth Calman, the then Chief Medical Officer (England), introduced these changes in a process known colloquially as 'Calmanization'.

Many feel that Calmanization has been responsible for disrupting the traditional structure of medical practice and apprentice-style training, particularly coupled as it was with health service reforms. It is more likely, however, that burgeoning financial pressures and increasing subspecialization, a direct consequence of medical progress, are more responsible for these changes. In fact, Calman's reforms have introduced a definite structure into training, previously a rather fragmented and haphazard affair, and the only real disadvantages are the somewhat short duration and relative inflexibility of the system.

Implications for the junior doctor

Because the time designated for completion of training is now stipulated and, in effect, has been shortened – by as much as 50% in some specialties – it is essential that training is of a sufficiently high standard to cover everything during this time. However, towards the end of their training, many trainees still feel a certain lack of confidence, regardless of the quality of their training, due to what they perceive to be a relative lack of experience because time is so short.

The deaneries, Royal Colleges and specialty associations are closely involved in 'training the trainers' – this can be time-consuming for trainers who are also expected to maintain the same high standard of clinical service. In some areas, courses are provided for trainees, particularly for the acquisition of specific skills; however, these courses are often expensive and new money has seldom been made available to cover such expenses. Finally, there is the age-old problem: consultants are often reluctant to change the way in which they work. Indeed, some are unable to do so because they already do so much in their average working day. In the future, consultants are likely to have a contractual obligation to train their juniors and perform regular appraisals and formal assessments.

be **actively involved** in your **training** from the **start**

There is a tendency for many trainees to be passive during the early years of their training and only to become actively concerned about the range and depth of their experience as the end of their training looms. They then become worried that they do not have sufficient experience and knowledge to take up a consultant appointment. Being actively involved in your training from the start will ensure you make the very best of your training and avoid this pitfall.

At the beginning of every attachment, sit down with the senior who has been designated your educational superior or 'trainer' (see page 14) and discuss your training needs from your own perspective as well as the opportunities of the post from their perspective. Periodically thereafter, perhaps every few months, discuss your progress with your seniors, from both your and their perspective, to ensure that you are constantly and progressively achieving your training goals. Accept any criticisms open-mindedly. Use them to focus on your weaker attributes so that you can improve them and become a better all-round doctor.

How to become a consultant

Courses versus practical experience

Courses are a valuable way of covering areas of subspecialty activity when 'hands-on' experience is unavailable, but trainees should aim for 'hands-on' experience whenever possible. If it is important to your training programme that such experience is made available, course attendance is simply a source of educational and theoretical reinforcement.

Organization of training

Training is organized by two broad groups of people, although there is a considerable degree of overlap.

Regional postgraduate deans

These men and women:
- are responsible for the employment and education of pre-registration house officers and senior house officers (i.e. those who have not yet chosen a specific career path)
- review, and are taking an increasing role in supervising, the progress of specialist registrars
- employ postgraduate clinical tutors who work in the postgraduate medical centres in all hospitals with trainees
- head the regional training committees, which liaise with the regional specialist training committees (STCs). These are responsible for the training in each recognized specialty within the region, a recognized specialty being one that has a specialist advisory committee (SAC) responsible to the appropriate Royal College.

Training in all specialties is organized as rotational programmes that last for 5 or 6 years. If the specialty is small, there may be only one training programme in a region. For larger specialties, such as general medicine or general surgery, several training programmes run concurrently in a region, and will all be subject to the regional STC. The chairman of each STC sits on the postgraduate dean's regional training committee at which matters relating to all specialties are discussed. Some specialties, such as cardiology, are particularly competitive; others, like obstetrics and gynaecology, have more trainees than there are consultant positions available at present.

Royal Colleges and specialist faculties

Through their various Joint Committees, the medical Royal Colleges and their specialist faculties organize the final professional examinations (e.g. MRCP, FRCS, MRCOG), and inspect and accredit training units for the purposes of training. To assist them, the colleges have advisors at local and regional levels: at a regional and national level, the SACs are responsible to the Joint Committees of Higher Medical Training (JCHMT) and Higher Surgical Training (JCHST) for their particular specialty. For each specialty, the regional STC provides the link between the postgraduate dean and the Royal College. In short, the Royal Colleges set the training standards and organize examinations at the end of the training period, while it is the responsibility of the postgraduate deans to ensure that standards are maintained.

The training process

Training begins with the 'basic professional training', the houseman year. Final-year students often agonize over their choice – or allocation – of house job; in reality, no one will pay much attention to your house job as long as you did it reasonably well. After basic professional training, specialist medical or surgical training begins with appointment as a senior house officer. The first stage is basic specialist training and at the end of this time – usually about 2 years – the initial professional examination (Part 1 MRCP in medicine, FRCS in surgery) is taken. The trainee often decides when this should be taken, but it should be a joint decision with his trainer. A pass is needed for the trainee to seek a place on a programme of higher medical or surgical training. Bear in mind that there are far more senior house officers than there are specialist registrar training posts to be filled. The number of specialist registrar posts

use your **senior house officer** post to **gain experience** in a **particular specialty**

How to become a consultant

available is tightly controlled and is falling in many specialties. Consequently, most aspiring specialists spend at least a year at the so-called senior house officer 3 level (i.e. they remain in a senior house officer grade although they have passed the relevant professional examination). As the senior house officer's post may be the first chance a trainee has to gain experience in a particular specialty, this opportunity should be welcomed and exploited to the full.

Getting a specialist registrar post

Designated training posts – specialist registrar posts – are advertised in the medical press; for most people, the traditional source of reference is the appointments section of the *BMJ*. Nowadays, almost all advertisements undergo careful scrutiny before they are finally published. The postgraduate deans have more or less imposed a standard advertisement, job specification and application form for all training posts. Unless you are fortunate enough to have another degree or previous work experience, research experience and any publications arising from it are the only relevant additional features that can score extra points in the highly competitive bid to be short-listed for interview.

Successful CVs

If you are required to apply with a CV, however, it is vitally important that it is accurately written, properly set out and well printed on good-quality white paper. Always ask a colleague to check it carefully, particularly for correct spelling and grammar. Avoid unusual fonts that may be more difficult to read – either Times or Arial is a good bet. For the sake of clarity, do not overuse upper-case letters or underlining; it is best not to use italic at all. A wide margin on the left-hand side will allow committee members to make notes. Four or five pages is probably the ideal length for a CV in application for a senior house officer's post.

Rather than simply listing your qualifications and previous positions, describe what you achieved from each of them and how they make you an excellent candidate for the position in question – this will increase your chances of success (Table 1). False modesty will prevent your CV from shining out from the rest!

Table 1

Compiling a CV: make the difference

Academic qualifications
- Emphasize any additional degrees or other qualifications you may have, and explain why these make you an attractive candidate for the post

Career statement
- Explain why you want the position on offer and why you are an excellent candidate
- Highlight your skills, such as communication, teaching, teamworking, information technology and audit

Employment history
- Only give full details relevant to the application
- Describe what you have gained from the positions, any unusual tasks undertaken and skills acquired
- Don't leave gaps – these generate suspicion. If, for example, you were travelling abroad for some time, say what you gained from this experience

Courses
- List all the courses you have attended, describing how you have benefited from them

Research
- Include research experience even if it is not a requirement; it is likely to count in your favour

Outside interests
- Don't include too many; you want to communicate that you are interesting, but not too busy. Be sure you can substantiate any claims!
- Include pursuits that demonstrate commitment and teamwork – don't just list reading and listening to music
- Try to convey the impression that you are an active rather than passive individual

How to become a consultant

Projecting yourself

Similarly, it is becoming more and more common for referees to provide a structured reference answering directed questions, rather than to submit one or two freehand paragraphs on the candidate's suitability for the job. Generally, a specialist registrar appointment committee will set out the key qualities desired; applications are scored against this checklist for short-listing and then again during the interview. As most applicants have very similar experience and very similar scores based on the objective evidence of the CV, this procedure is designed to identify the person who stands out and will presumably be the best candidate for the position. It is therefore particularly important to project yourself well during the interview (Table 2).

Table 2

Strategy for the training-post interview

- Visit the unit in advance, see as many relevant people as possible and gather all the information you can about the post
- Prepare answers to likely questions – a dummy run with your current trainer might be particularly helpful in this respect
- Arrive in plenty of time for the interview (at least 20 minutes in advance) looking keen, professional and presentable

During the interview
- Sit upright and try to look keen and enthusiastic, yet confident and relaxed – try to avoid appearing overconfident or too laid back
- Answer the questions directly, looking at the questioner – don't ramble on, just stick to the point
- Focus on and convey eloquently the reasons why you are the ideal candidate for the job and emphasize the skills you can bring to the unit
- At the end of the interview, you may be asked if you have any questions – prepare one that makes it clear that you are very keen on the job and enthusiastic about the unit and the hospital

---

Specialist registrar grade

Successful applicants to the specialist registrar grade will be awarded a 'number' by the specialist training committee acting on behalf of the regional postgraduate dean. For those individuals who have the right of permanent domicile in the UK, and who are therefore undergoing so-called 'type-1' training, this will be a national training number (NTN). Type-1 training ultimately leads to the award of a Certificate of Completion of Specialist Training (CCST), with which the trainee can apply to the Specialist Training Authority for entry onto the specialist register. This, in turn, allows him to apply for a consultant appointment. Thus the CCST is the all-important goal if you are aiming to be a consultant in the UK.

For those successful applicants who do not have the right of domicile in the UK, a visiting training number (VTN) and so-called 'type-2' training, which does not lead to a CCST, are given. Type-2 trainees are awarded a certificate to show that they have completed a programme of training. They may also take the relevant professional examination for their specialty, for which, if they pass, they will receive a further certificate. They cannot, however, be entered onto the specialist register as a specialist in the UK.

At the time of your successful interview or shortly thereafter, you will discuss whether you have any previous accreditable training with the postgraduate dean. If you do not, your CCST date (UK trainees only) will usually be set at a point 5 or 6 years, depending on the specialty, after the date on which you take up your new appointment as a specialist registrar.

Previous accreditable experience

Previous accreditable experience is generally up to 1 year spent in research, although some other experience may be accreditable under certain circumstances, subject to specific rules and regulations. For example, a period as a locum is accreditable if it is classified as time spent in a 'locum appointment for training' (LAT). If it is deemed unsuitable as a LAT, it will be designated a 'locum appointment for service' (LAS), which is not accreditable. A LAT should have prospective approval for time that can be counted against type-1 or type-2 training when that individual is subsequently appointed as a specialist registrar. Likewise, time in a fixed-term training appointment (FTTA) can count towards training if it meets certain prospectively determined criteria. Time spent in a LAS post cannot count towards a CCST, however valuable it may be otherwise in terms of experience.

On appointment

At the time of appointment, an initial record of in-training assessment (RITA) form is completed by the regional STC acting on behalf of the postgraduate dean. This will summarize your experience to date, including any previous accreditable time and, taking these into account, your projected CCST date. Your progress is recorded annually, using the RITA system, by the STC acting on behalf of the regional postgraduate dean. Satisfactory progress attracts one type of RITA form, unsatisfactory progress another. Subject to satisfactory progress, your trainer will recommend you to the SAC for that specialty shortly before your CCST date arrives and when, if you are a surgical trainee, you have passed the final professional examination. The SAC then recommends through the appropriate Royal College committee that they, in turn, recommend the award of CCST and eventual registration on the Specialist Register.

All higher specialist training must be in recognized training posts in recognized training units and in recognized training programmes. Accreditation of these posts, units and programmes is the responsibility of the SAC, but this is being conducted with the increasing involvement of postgraduate deans through the joint auspices of the STCs.

Assessment

Having understood the process involved, the next step as an aspiring specialist is to understand what is required of you. There will be a curriculum of training or 'educational contract', a syllabus for the final professional examination (for surgical trainees) and a list of skills required for your chosen specialty. Be sure to know what is required of you in each of these regards and whether you need to acquire them in any particular order or at any specific stage of your training.

know what is **required** of **you** and **plan** your **progress**

Strictly speaking, assessment is the formal process by which a trainee's progress is measured against established criteria. At the very least, this includes passing the examination at the end of training if you are in a surgical specialty. Annual assessment by the regional STC, culminating in the issue of the appropriate RITA form, incorporates, at least theoretically, the setting of interim goals to be achieved and measures progress against these goals in all specialties.

Find out from your trainer about compulsory and voluntary courses for skills acquisition. Then find out about annual assessments and how they are conducted. Your programme director or current trainer will tell you how this operates in theory, but other trainees will tell you what actually happens in practice. Very often, you will have to plan yourself how to acquire the necessary expertise year by year.

The most important step is to find a mentor – a 'trainer' who is willing and able to give not only advice and support but also feedback on your progress. Ideally, all trainers should be mentors for the duration of your time together, but in practice some trainers are more enthusiastic and approachable than others. It is important that your trainer is someone who you get along with, can talk openly to and who will actively offer you help and tell you if you are on the wrong track. Postgraduate deans have systems in place for dealing with people who fail to achieve their targets, but it is very important that you are made aware of any potential problems by your trainer, programme director or mentor long before that stage is reached. Of course, it is your responsibility to know your own targets and eventual goals.

A good relationship with a designated trainer is the best way of getting advice and feedback. Ideally, you will receive constructive feedback from each of your trainers during your training. All too often, however, even when there is a good relationship between trainee and trainer, the trainee just slips into a job at the beginning and out again at the end without being aware of what he should have learnt or whether, in fact, he has learnt it. Make time to meet and talk during your training. If your trainer is not willing to give you his time, find someone who will.

Appraisal

Appraisal, on the other hand, is the informal process in which the trainee and trainer agree objectives for a training period (usually 1 year), the goal being to achieve a satisfactory assessment by the STC at the end of that period. Thus, at the beginning of your training period, you and your trainer should meet to discuss what is expected of you, agreeing measurable targets and appropriate interim goals.

Mock appraisal document

Today, I met with Joe Bloggs at the start of his 1-year attachment to this unit. He is a second-year specialist registrar and spent the last year working at Anywhere District General Hospital where he says he received a good grounding in the specialty. Prior to this, he completed his basic training at St Elsewhere's. In between basic training and higher training, he did a year in research, which went well and provided him with some good and interesting results, though he is yet to write up the project and submit it to the *Journal of Clinical Appropriateness*.

We discussed the timetable for his current post and identified the following goals.

1. He needs to learn the technique of exploratory pharyngoscopy.
2. He needs some exposure to advanced pharyngoscopic techniques as he has not encountered these in his general training so far.
3. He needs to attend a course on cardiopulmonary resuscitation, which is a fundamental training requirement, and should also attend the annual scientific meeting of the British Association of Exploratory Pharyngoscopists.
4. He should write up his paper and aim to submit it by the time of his 6-monthly review.

We have agreed to meet again in 6 months when the above issues will form the agenda for the next appraisal meeting. Also, an assessment of his clinical progress by that stage will be made and we will discuss where he ought to go on the next leg of the rotation.

Signed by the both of us.

_____   _____

Date: _____   Date: _____

It is the responsibility of your trainer to document all appraisals properly. You should both agree an agenda for your appraisal, preferably a standard agenda for all trainees, and then adhere to it. Points discussed should be noted, and both you and your trainer should sign and keep a copy of the document; this will act as the agenda for the next appraisal meeting. Likewise, all assessments should be documented and signed by both parties. A signature does not indicate that the party agrees with the entire content of the document – it merely confirms that the document is a true representation of the topics discussed and opinions expressed. The appraisal system is an important way of ensuring that goals are achieved in training and that the necessary skills are acquired.

The final examination for surgical trainees

Although the end of the training period is fixed by the date of the CCST and is therefore simply a matter of time, the definitive hurdle for most surgical trainees and many other specialties is the final professional examination. Each specialty with a SAC has its own intercollegiate examination, which takes many different forms. The tendency is to move away from essays and short-answer questions coupled with clinical examinations and vivas to more objective assessments, such as multiple-choice questions and objective, structured clinical examinations (OSCEs). In the surgical specialties, interest is developing in the objective, structured assessment of technical skills (OSATS). Currently used in Canada, OSATS is being piloted in some surgical specialties in the UK. Log books and other portfolios of practical experience are also important, particularly in surgical and other specialties, such as gastroenterology, radiology and nephrology, in which interventional techniques are important. In some instances, published papers or case reviews must be submitted.

the **aim** of **exams** is to **show you** are **safe** and **competent**

According to most examiners, the examinations are not particularly difficult. Indeed, in the past, few examinees have found them to be a struggle. Most examiners seek only to ensure that the examinee is safe and competent – they are not looking to find a potential candidate for

How to become a consultant

the next Nobel prize in medicine. However, as the training period has become shortened and, as a result, more intensive, pressure has mounted on candidates to pass because, in theory, they could be out of a job if they keep on failing, so anxiety levels among examinees have risen. Unsurprisingly, the failure rate has also risen in some specialties. All too often, candidates find that they become nervous and anxious, and consequently make silly mistakes. However, there are a number of positive steps that can be taken to maximize your chances (Table 3).

Table 3

Passing the final examination in surgery

Planning your examination
- Take your examination at the earliest possible opportunity so that the pressure of time is less – assuming of course that you are likely to pass

Preparation
- Digest articles from review journals, rather than textbooks, such as those in the *Current Opinion* and *Clinics of North America* series (these are good sources of general information that will help you to satisfy the examiner that you are safe and competent)
- Ensure that you have some practice of whatever form the final examination will take. Some specialties have in-service examinations as part of their annual training and assessment cycle or, alternatively, any of the numerous books of multiple-choice questions available in each specialty may be helpful
- Revise adequately, don't just hope for the best and 'wing it'

On the day
- Go outside for a walk between vivas or papers
- Try to stay away from other candidates – they will just make you more nervous

---

Subspecialization

The general rule in medical specialties is to be trained in general internal medicine plus a specialty. In the case of surgery, general training ceases after basic surgical training and all subsequent training is within the specialty. But in both circumstances, many trainees will want to pursue a particular subspecialty interest. This is usually done at the end of training, after the final professional examination has been passed but before the CCST date. It is important to plan this as far in advance as possible. Obviously it is difficult to do this when it is contingent on the outcome of an examination or some other process. However, competition for these subspecialist training posts can be fierce, and you must ensure that you do not lose the job by failing to notify the trainer or programme director of your interest in sufficient time.

At the moment, subspecialty training is informal, with no particular entry or exit criteria. In due course, it is likely that if you undergo subspecialty training, you will need to accrue a portfolio of experience and satisfy some type of assessment to show that you have reached an appropriate standard in advanced medical or surgical care in that particular area. It is also very likely that such documentation will become an essential part of the selection criteria for subspecialty posts at consultant grade. So, for example, you will not be able to perform 'switch' operations as a paediatric cardiac surgeon until you have some form of certification to show that you have been trained to do them and have attained an adequate level of competence.

Flexible training

Flexible training has been introduced for those who find it difficult, if not impossible, to work full-time. This training method is primarily aimed at women with young children, but anyone with a well-founded reason, be it domestic commitments, disability or ill health, for feeling unable to work full-time can be considered.

Candidates must first be appointed to a specialist registrar post in open competition. Only then can they apply to the postgraduate dean for flexible training. Each dean's office will have someone responsible for flexible training.

Specialist registrars are expected to work a minimum of five sessions per week – in other words, at least half time – with an appropriate on-call duty. Overall, they are expected to spend the same amount of time in training as those in the full-time programme. So if full-time training takes 6 years, a specialist registrar working 50% of the time would be in training for 12 years. Specialist registrars can change from part- to full-time training, and can also change regions, as their circumstances alter.

Duties of a doctor: GMC guidelines

At the end of your training, you should feel sufficiently confident to make the next step to becoming a consultant. At all times, remember and adhere to the guidelines set by the GMC.

Duties of a doctor

Patients must be able to trust doctors with their lives and well-being. To justify that trust, we as a profession have a duty to maintain a good standard of practice and care and to show respect for human life.

In particular, as a doctor you must:

- make the care of the patient your first concern
- treat every patient politely and considerately
- respect patients' dignity and privacy
- listen to patients and respect their views
- give patients information in a way they can understand
- respect the rights of patients to be fully involved in decisions about their care
- keep your professional knowledge and skills up to date
- recognise the limits of your professional competence
- be honest and trustworthy
- respect and protect confidential information
- make sure that your personal beliefs do not prejudice your patients' care
- act quickly to protect patients from risk if you have good reason to believe that you or a colleague may not be fit to practice
- avoid abusing your position as a doctor
- work with colleagues in the ways' that best serve your patients' interests.

In all these matters, you must never discriminate unfairly against your patients or colleagues. And you must always be prepared to justify your actions to them.

Reproduced from *Good Medical Practice*. London: GMC, 1998.

Further reading

Downie RS, Macnaughton J. *Clinical Judgement: Evidence in Practice.* Oxford: Oxford University Press, 2000.

Eggert M. *The Perfect Interview – All You Need to Get it Right First Time.* London: Century, 1992.

Gatrell J, White T. *The Specialist Registrar Handbook.* Abingdon: Radcliffe Medical Press, 1999.

General Medical Council. *Good Medical Practice.* London: GMC, 1998.

O'Brien E. Prepare a curriculum vitae. In: *How to Do It.* Vol 2. London: BMJ, 1985.

How to become a consultant

research

"Where observation is concerned, chance favours only the prepared mind"
Louis Pasteur 1822–95

At trainee level

A few trainees undertake research because they genuinely want to conduct experimental or clinical studies to find out more about, or make a breakthrough in, a particular subject. These folk, unfortunately, are rather rare. In reality, research is more often performed to enhance a CV or because an individual feels unable to refuse a keen consultant. Time in research is valuable, however, not only in terms of improving your CV. You will gain experience in searching the literature, assessing conflicting results and opinions, and interpreting what you read. You will also learn scientific methodology and the use of particular techniques – having first-hand experience inevitably makes it easier to assess the results of others. And of course, you will also have the opportunity to have papers published in peer-reviewed journals and to present your work at national and international meetings. This time can also be used to develop your ability to think strategically and manage your time effectively.

Defining your research

The first step is to decide the research you want to perform. Be clear about the objectives of your proposed research. Next, read around the subject carefully to find out whether the research has been done previously – this will also help you focus on the work you intend to do. It is particularly important to find a supervisor who will oversee your project from start to finish and ensure that you benefit from your research experience. If you are not in the right place with the right people and the right facilities, then you may have to go elsewhere or modify your plans to fit the location.

Profile of a good supervisor

A good supervisor:
- is interested in what you are doing
- has the time and inclination to help you to do it
- has facilities at his disposal and is able to draw on the expertise of others to help in areas where he cannot help you himself or at times when he is unavailable
- will say what he thinks without equivocation and give useful advice and direction
- will check your written work carefully, correct it and provide further guidance when necessary
- will motivate you to complete the project

Prepare a written proposal or protocol for your intended research. This should include:
- a critical review of the literature to date – use this to justify your study
- a reasonably detailed outline of the proposed study – what is your research goal and how are you going to achieve it?
- plans for the statistical methodology that you are going to use to interpret your results.

If the work involves human subjects and impacts on patients, you will need to submit your proposal to an ethical committee or to the Trust's research committee for approval and/or to funding bodies. For all practical purposes, all research must be submitted to an ethical committee for approval, but even if a proposal is not needed for the above reasons, this preparation will focus your thoughts and help you to explain your proposal to others, particularly your supervisor. When you have finished your first draft, scrutinize it and improve it if at all possible. Give it to a colleague, whose opinion you value and respect, to read.

You should then obtain an expert opinion and appropriate statistical guidance from your supervisor. Most hospitals have a statistics expert available who will be able to help you to ensure that your study has the best possible chance of producing meaningful results. Nowadays, there are many good statistical software packages available. When you have a supervisor-approved protocol, you can submit it to the appropriate bodies. Bear in mind that they may want revisions made and may even turn down a revised proposal. Nonetheless, if you have a good supervisor, you should be able to get it right eventually.

Getting started

There is often a phase between submission of a grant or ethical committee application and receiving a reply when it appears that there is nothing much to do. Actually there is quite a lot to do. In particular, this time may be used for reading to ensure that, when your experimental study begins, the majority of background reading has been done.

If it is a clinical study then you can begin to recruit patients, which is always more difficult and time-consuming than you think it will be at the outset, irrespective of your subject. Patients can be identified and approached informally before an ethics committee has given formal approval. If it is laboratory research, then you can start to familiarize yourself with instrumentation, either directly or by watching others work. Time is the most valuable commodity in research – do not waste it!

Practical points

When you perform your research, whether a clinical study or laboratory investigation, make sure everybody concerned knows what you are doing. You may need help and advice, and you will certainly not want to be forgotten! Try to integrate yourself into the team.

As you work, it is important to document all you do – make duplicate copies whenever you can and back up computer files on to disks regularly. If possible, obtain a laptop computer and install software for compiling references. Equally important, start to write up your project at the earliest possible opportunity as it always takes longer than you think. When you are not actively researching,

never waste time during **research**

write. All too often, research is completed before writing up begins: the funding runs out and the researcher takes a clinical job and no longer has the time to write up. It is tragic to contemplate how much good-quality research never sees the light of day for this reason, and the number of careers that are marred by the failure to deliver the results of their research.

At a more senior level

Senior research is a serious business that requires serious money. Whereas at trainee level, a first project is likely to be a case review or review of the literature surrounding an interesting clinical observation, research at a more senior, advanced level requires a substantial amount of new work. The expense of starting a new study and the uncertainties of funding are such that research is always best carried out in a department with a track record in that particular area, in which equipment, expertise and a considerable volume of experience already exist.

Getting funding

The principal difficulty with research at this level is funding. Research departments exist on the grant income that they raise both directly and indirectly. Directly, a grant will pay the salaries of most of the people who work in the department, apart from the fortunate, but increasingly rare, senior scientists with tenured appointments that are funded by the department until they retire. Indirectly, the level and source of funding constitute the means by which university department review committees assess research departments, such as the Research Assessment Exercise (RAE) conducted by the Higher Education Funding Council for England (HEFCE). A £50 000 grant from the Medical Research Council (MRC) or the Wellcome Trust (awarded after a competitive peer-review process) may be considered by the RAE to be more prestigious than £100 000 from an anonymous private donor.

apply to a **funding body** with a **tradition** of **supporting work** in your **field**

The first step is to decide whether the research to be undertaken is of sufficient scientific merit to attract the interest of one of the major grant-giving bodies. If so, the next step is to approach the most appropriate grant-giving body, or bodies, and obtain a copy of their instructions to applicants, which will outline the procedure and timing for applications. Many of the larger funding bodies also issue annual reports that list the organization's research priorities – you should be able to find out whether your planned research is in one of the areas generally funded by that body. Some bodies also welcome informal applications to discuss a proposal before formal submission.

Clinical research

The main source of funding for clinically orientated research is the NHS Research and Development Initiative, the principal aim of which is to develop the database necessary for sound decisions on health policy. Health Technology Assessment is the largest of the programmes within this initiative, and its research priorities are identified and published by the Standing Group on Health Technology.

Laboratory-based research

The leading body for funding laboratory research (although also involved in health services research) is the MRC. It provides a wide range of grants, not only for individual studies, but also for training fellowships and travel grants for work in overseas departments. Anyone considering a period in research before becoming a consultant should consider a training fellowship, particularly if you intend to continue your career as a consultant in academic medicine or surgery. The MRC publishes its research priorities widely and clearly, but is particularly interested in collaborative applications, preferably from several institutions conducting large-scale multidisciplinary research. For non-cancer-related research, the Wellcome Trust is the other major funding body. It tends to be less molecular-biology orientated and encourages informal approaches in the first instance to verify whether formal applications are appropriate. Otherwise it functions in much the same way as the MRC.

Cancer research is supported mainly by the Cancer Research Campaign and the Imperial Cancer Research Fund, both of which favour multidisciplinary collaborative research. There is a number of other large charities that concentrate on specific diseases, such as the British Heart Foundation, the Arthritis and Rheumatism Council and the National Kidney Research Fund. Each of these, like the MRC, offers several different types of grant. A list of charities that fund medical research in relation to particular diseases outside of these areas can be found in the

Association of Medical Research Charities Handbook (see *Useful addresses*, page 171).

European funding
The European Commission is becoming increasingly important in funding research. It includes a European Community Research and Development Programme, comparable to the NHS Research and Development Initiative, and an Economic and Social Research Council, comparable to the MRC, although its primary fields of interest are psychology- and sociology-based studies.

Non-medical funding bodies
There are research councils, other than the MRC, relevant to those in medical research, particularly in biomaterials or biotechnology. Organizations such as the Engineering and Physical Sciences Research Council (EPSRC) and the Biotechnology and Biological Sciences Research Council (BBSRC) function in much the same way as the MRC and produce their own handbooks outlining the grants and awards available. The Department of Trade and Industry funds six LINK programmes in healthcare to promote collaboration between university departments and industry. These are particularly appropriate for those engaged in research which is likely to produce new technology that has the potential to be developed commercially by the industrial partner. Many smaller charities also offer grants for research focused on their own area of interest.

Types of grant

The most common type of grant from these bodies is the project grant. A project grant is designed to support a specific study by covering the salary of a full-time research assistant for 2–3 years, together with the costs of the research study itself in terms of equipment and consumables. Such grants run to tens of thousands of pounds.

Rather more prestigious is a programme grant that covers the cost of a large-scale study by supporting a research team and its associated costs rather than just an individual. These often run to hundreds of thousands of pounds. Very few of these grants are awarded each year and it is the pinnacle of a researcher's ambition to receive one – an award deemed only slightly lower than winning a Nobel Prize! Only a team of experienced researchers could expect to receive a programme grant. The value of training fellowships and their importance to the developing academic should not be underestimated. Finally, project grants in which a relatively small amount of money is awarded are sometimes available for pilot studies of short duration.

Grant applications

All grants are awarded after intense competitive scrutiny. Grant application writing is an arduous process (many universities have departments dedicated to helping researchers produce grant applications) and most applications submitted are likely to be rejected. The principles are the same as those for preparing an outline proposal at a junior level, but should be applied much more rigorously. The application must outline the purpose of the study. The need for new research into this area should be supported by a brief literature review. The aims must be clearly outlined, indicating the potential benefits of the study, followed by a full description of the intended methodology, including data to be collected and statistical techniques for analysis. Study requirements must then be stated and justified in detail. These will include salaries for research staff, essential equipment and running costs, including consumables, and other expenses such as travel and subsistence to present research results. Funding bodies usually, but not always, have a specific application form to present this information, although some like the Wellcome Trust prefer an informal written approach, in the first instance; they will forward an application form if the proposal is of interest.

All funding bodies have a similar assessment process to deal with applications. They have a grants committee that includes their own experts and external referees with expertise in the particular subject area to review applications. At least two, and often more, external referees will review and individually rate each application. A group of applications will then be considered together by the committee.

> **success** hinges on a **well-prepared, clear** and **concise application**

Competition is such that all applications are likely to be of an extremely high standard, so only those with an alpha plus or similar rating from the internal and external referees are likely to be accepted, and even these cannot assume success.

Each applicant, therefore, needs to convince the reviewers that his application poses an important research question, will use appropriate and feasible research methodology, and if possible that the study will be conducted by researchers with experience in that particular area. Commonly, applications are unsuccessful because the research question is unimportant and/or poorly presented, or the research methodology or analytical techniques are inappropriate or imprecise. Occasionally, there may be insufficient experience or expertise in the research team to bring the research to a satisfactory conclusion.

The key to success is a well-prepared, clear and concise application. If a previous application has been submitted or if preliminary advice has been sought from the funding body, take notice of any criticisms and comments, and ensure that the application is put together carefully, allowing plenty of time to write, rewrite and rewrite again if necessary. Follow the application instructions supplied by the funding body closely and seek advice from those with experience in writing grant applications. Read through the application in detail and remove any excess or inappropriate text. Most important of all, don't be surprised or disappointed if your first application is turned down. Writing a successful grant application is an academic goal in its own right.

Alternative funding bodies

There are other, albeit less prestigious, sources of funding for research. The most widely used are the local charities affiliated to hospital Trusts. Similar application procedures apply, but generally these are less formal although still rigorous. Professional societies such as the Royal Colleges have funds available for research grants, often in the form of fellowships, which are only marginally less prestigious than those from the major grant-giving bodies.

Most major drug companies and medical equipment manufacturers sponsor medical research. Indeed, in the UK, pharmaceutical company-sponsored research overall is currently the largest contributor to medical research. Much of this 'soft money' is dedicated to the development and marketing of new drugs, but some may be awarded as a fellowship for more altruistic purposes, in which case similar application procedures will apply. Getting these grants is often quicker and easier than going through the traditional funding bodies. When submitting a proposal for such a grant, remember the 'What's in it for them?' principle. Pharmaceutical companies are businesses and are unlikely to sponsor projects that do not reflect the general direction in which they are heading. Be sure that the work you perform for them, and others, always maintains the highest ethical standards.

Writing up

The principles involved in writing a thesis or preparing a paper for publication in a journal are essentially the same. In the first instance, you should decide for whom you are writing and find out what rules and regulations apply. These are available from universities in the case of theses or from the journal to which you intend to submit your paper. The general format is an initial summary followed by an introduction, materials and methods, results and discussion sections. For a thesis, the introduction is usually a detailed historical literature review of the general subject together with an outline of the question under

> **write** up as you go **along** and **give drafts** to a **colleague** to **read**

consideration and another detailed relevant literature review specific to the study question. Whatever the nature of your publication, it will be reviewed by at least two experts in the field who will be familiar with, and may well have contributed to, the relevant literature. They will be aware of the difficulties that exist in your particular area of research and will expect to see adequate coverage of the potential sources of error in your study in the discussion section. Equally important to a critical analysis of potential sources of error is the future relevance of any research findings. Which questions remain unanswered and where should future research be directed to develop further the implications of your study?

Aim to have as much as possible written up before completing your research, though data analysis will need to wait until all the results are available. Write as you go along and as soon as you have finished a first draft, give it to somebody else to read. Expect them to tear it to shreds – this is all part of the learning process. Use this criticism constructively; it is preferable for your supervisor to point out defects in your work in private than for an examiner or an audience to do so during a viva or at a major national or international meeting. Such criticism should not be taken as a personal insult but instead viewed as positive feedback.

Remember that when you have completed a piece of research you will automatically be one of the world's leading authorities on that very narrow topic. Indeed, unless you have simply repeated somebody else's specific investigation, you will be *the* leading authority on the subject, at least for a brief time. Therefore, others will criticize you (in the strictest sense of the word) not so much about *what* you have done but on *how* you have done it. The most important part of published research, to the critical reader, is the critical self-analysis in the discussion section. Analyse all potential sources of error in the conclusions you have derived from your results, particularly with reference to methodology. When examining your thesis, the examiner will probably concentrate on how you have critically reviewed the literature in the first chapter and your analysis of results in the discussion section later on. Your results – although probably dearest to your heart – will often be less important to the examiner than your interpretation of them.

Statistical work, particularly involving clinical evaluation of patients, should be presented very carefully and reviewed following guidelines such as those laid down in the *BMJ*. Statistical advice should have been sought before the project began to ensure that no problems would come to light at this late stage. In short, research involves a great deal of work, but most people appreciate it or learn something from it, and hopefully both.

Supervising a research project

If you are supervising a research project that is being conducted by others, you should aim to fulfil the criteria that you expected of your supervisor when you were the junior partner. It is a good idea to hold weekly meetings at which every researcher in the team presents their results and progress to date, and that provide an opportunity for constructive critical appraisal by colleagues. In addition, meet with each researcher to discuss his work to date and monitor progress against the project timetable that has been set within the constraints of time and funding. In particular, ensure that the research is written up and that each draft is handed to you to read through; give constructive criticism and comments, and set a deadline for submission of each revised draft until you are satisfied with the final copy.

Finally, identify any interesting ideas for future research so that, if possible, these can be developed by a subsequent researcher. You are likely to be acknowledged in his publications and you may be able to maintain valuable long-term contact with the institution.

Pharmaceutical company-sponsored projects

The pharmaceutical industry is the main source of research funding in the UK overall. Unlike the major grant-giving bodies and private donors who normally respond to a research proposal, pharmaceutical companies direct the research they sponsor and the researcher's responsibility is to manage the project. In most instances, the pharmaceutical company will determine the objectives of the study although there is sometimes opportunity for discussion of the details. Indeed, you are likely to have been approached because of your particular expertise in the field.

It is important not to underestimate the financial value of your research in pharmaceutical company-sponsored projects, nor to overestimate its intellectual value. In any project, most of the benefit comes from planning the patient selection methodology and, in particular, the statistical assessment and analysis of results. In research sponsored by pharmaceutical companies, they usually perform the analysis when data from individual patient studies are sent back to them. Carefully consider the time that you will need to invest before embarking on such a project. Before committing yourself, ask around to find out the going rate so that you are in a position to negotiate and ensure that you are not undervalued. However, be aware that there is intense financial pressure to generate results.

If you do take part in clinical trials, or indeed any other research enlisting patients or volunteers, you are responsible for ensuring that each patient understands the implications, has given written, informed consent for his involvement in the trial, and that the research is not contrary to his interests. You should always seek further advice in cases where individuals are not able to make decisions for themselves and, in particular, if undertaking research that involves children. Always be sure to check that a properly constituted research ethics committee has approved the research protocol.

Further reading

Association of Medical Research Charities Handbook. London: AMRC, 2000.

Baxter L, Hughes C, Tight M. *How to Research.* Buckingham: Open University Press, 1996.

Benatar D, Benatar SR. Informed consent and research. *BMJ* 1998;316:1008.

Murrell G, Huang C, Ellis H. *Research in Medicine: Planning a Project – Writing a Thesis.* 2nd edn. Cambridge: Cambridge University Press, 1999.

Power L. Trial subjects must be fully involved in design and approval of trials. *BMJ* 1998;316:1003–4.

Sieber JE. *Planning Ethically Responsible Research.* London: Sage Publications, 1992.

the NHS:
making your mark

"Seek opportunity, not security. A boat in a harbour is safe, but in time its bottom will rot out"
H Jackson Brown Jr in *Life's Little Instruction Book*

So your post is secured. You have reached the first real post-qualification high point – you are a consultant. But beware! This is the point at which many doctors find themselves becoming somewhat disillusioned. With no obvious goals to achieve, many experience a form of anxiety or depression. So, how can you maintain and build on your initial success?

Striving for continued success

Others (generally statutory bodies) have set the goals that you have achieved to date, but now you should begin to set your own goals. Indeed, setting and attaining personal goals is fundamental to your success as a consultant in the NHS – or indeed in any walk of life.

You must also appreciate the importance of change in clinical practice as well as in everyday life. Now that you no longer have examinations and superiors to make sure you develop, you yourself will have to seek out reasons to modify your practices and take responsibility for making the necessary improvements. Most importantly, do not allow yourself to become complacent and get left behind.

The last general point concerns your life outside medicine. Non-medical partners or spouses tend to assume that when you get to the top of the ladder – that is, become a consultant – you will not have to work so hard: your on-call duties will diminish, you will not have to stay late in the hospital every evening and so on. But you do not have to be a consultant for very long to know that this is patently untrue. In some instances, you will spend less time on call, but even so, this extra time will be more than compensated for by the enormous amount of extra paperwork, management and general clinical responsibility that a consultant takes on as the leader, or one of the leaders, of a clinical team. It is important then to remember your family and, in particular, that nobody on their deathbed ever says, 'I wish I had spent more time at work'. Look after yourself and your family – you should take care of your own health and your family's general well-being, and not allow yourself to become estranged from your friends and loved ones. Try to find a focus for your free time, ideally something that you can share with your family. There is nothing quite so boring as a consultant who comes home and buries himself in his papers and talks about nothing but work. For goodness' sake, avoid this at all costs! Achieving personal happiness and maintaining quality family relationships are equally as important as building a successful career, if not more so.

This is clearly not the place to tell readers how to achieve personal and family happiness; nor are the authors best placed to define this. However, it is worth mentioning that divorce is more common in medicine than in many other walks of life. Most doctors know of colleagues who have got into 'difficulties' trying to balance the competing demands of a medical career and a family. As with all aspects of life, it is easier to find a way through if you anticipate and talk about the problems, rather than sweeping them under the carpet or dealing with them when it is already too late.

balance your life – don't neglect personal relationships

Women, however, have the added difficulty of fitting childbearing around their training. In the past, many women who wished to have a family used to wait until they had become consultants before having children. Nowadays, it is more usual to elect to have 'flexible training', allowing training and motherhood to run concurrently. Deaneries have a designated flexible training coordinator to provide advice on such matters. Training committees should be sympathetic to the aspirations of *all* trainees – men as well as women – who want to undergo flexible training. Regardless of the stage at which children appear, they need to be incorporated into the 'grand plan' and that is, as always, best considered in advance.

Finding your focus

The single largest problem when finding your focus, setting goals and yet maintaining a healthy and rewarding life outside medicine is time. Generally, the most successful people are those who manage their time most effectively (see pages 37–9). Furthermore, because medicine involves dealing with people, either as patients or colleagues, successful individuals relate well to other people, often enlisting the help of others to enable them to use their time efficiently. The successful consultant knows what he is going to do and how he is going to do it; he sets himself objectives towards a final goal (and then maybe a further goal when that one has been achieved). Making the best of time and people usually means building a good team that functions efficiently.

Taking control

As a new consultant, the first thing you must do is determine how you will fulfil your contractual obligation of fixed and flexible sessions, and on-call commitments. These vary from post to post, and will be clearly stated in the job description. Then, you must establish how you are going to carry out your clinical practice, fulfil any teaching commitments and conduct any planned research. Other aspects to consider include:

- establishing and running your own office
- developing a good working relationship with your secretary
- ensuring that you have sufficient junior staff and equipment.

Of these, an efficient secretary and office are particularly important. Equipment and trainees are usually provided or allocated by other agencies, but establishing an efficient office with a good secretary is very much a personal concern. It is important to establish a routine so that people know what you do and when, and instances when you can or cannot be interrupted or contacted. Allow yourself a protected time during the week to think, plan, reflect, and deal with paperwork and other routine management issues. Also, set aside time for informal discussion and let your colleagues know when you will be available.

At this stage, it is helpful to obtain advice, whether you feel you need it or not, from others who have been through the same experience already. What do they do and how do they do it? It is certainly not a weakness to ask for opinions and advice, and learning from the experience of others can save a great deal of time and prevent mistakes. Reading this book, of course, is a step in the right direction!

Increasing your clinical expertise

On a clinical level, it is important to keep up to date with your specialty not only by reading, but also by discussing clinical problems you encounter with the people you regard as your peers or those with greater expertise than yourself. The smaller your focus of interest becomes, the more difficult this may be. It has been said that experience allows you to recognize a mistake the next time you make it (and also that good judgement is the result of experience which is the result of bad judgement), but you can also learn from the mistakes of others.

Make sure that those you would like to regard as your peers are aware of your particular interest, and try to establish yourself as an authority in that area. Attend seminars and conferences in your chosen field – show your face and stand up to speak at appropriate opportunities to underline your interest. Publish as much as you can in that area, making sure that your publications are of the highest quality and relevant to others.

Keeping up to date

Some doctors become dissatisfied with medicine for a number of reasons: too much work and not enough time to do it; a declining income in real terms (as they see it); increasing medicolegal liability; anger, frustration, depression and a feeling of loss of control of their job and future. The issue most commonly cited, however, is information overload. There is simply too much being published and too much to know. It has been aptly said, 'We are drowning in information, but thirsting for knowledge.' Dealing with the volume of information and retrieving what you need to know is an essential skill you will need to acquire.

The first step is to think about how this applies to you. Time spent planning and reflecting is always valuable; decide what you need to know, where it can be found and how you are going to learn it or otherwise have it available. It is impossible to keep up to date with everything, so deciding what you actually need to know is vital.

Most people have piles of journals and unread material littered around their office and home. It usually remains unread because most of it does not need to be read. So establish what needs to be read, photocopy it or otherwise file it, and discard the journal. Having copied or filed it, electronically (an excellent option if you have access to a flat-bed scanner) or otherwise, make sure that you can retrieve it readily when necessary. Learning to use modern information technology is particularly valuable in this regard. Online journal databases provide a useful means of keeping up to date on subjects that you need to know about while avoiding irrelevant subjects. Purchase a personal laptop computer and learn to surf the Internet. Throughout your medical training and subsequent career, focus on your own continuing professional development, attitudes and interpersonal skills, and appraise them constantly. These are just as important as the more traditional scientific skills and knowledge.

Managing your time

It has been estimated that 80% of a person's productivity is a result of 20% of his time. If true, this means that most of our time is wasted. Some people are perfectionists and will achieve less because of their quest for perfection in everything they do. On balance, efficiency is better than perfection for most purposes, and becomes all the more important as your workload increases.

Set priorities, paying particular attention to tasks that only you can perform, and adhere to them. One of the most important management skills to acquire is successful delegation. If someone else could do a task as well, if not better, than you, then delegate it.

To use your time efficiently, never start something that you are not going to finish, and always complete one task before moving on to the next. Don't postpone an

efficiency is better than perfection

unpleasant or boring task – it will never improve with time – but do avoid starting anything when you are bored, depressed, tired or simply unable to focus and put in the effort required.

You should also think about the bigger picture and spend time developing your own personal strategy. Decide what your goals are and set yourself a realistic time-frame within which to achieve them. Carefully consider the potential pitfalls and identify what your key focus areas should be. Regularly, take the time to think about your strategy and constantly modify it as individual goals are achieved.

Paperwork

Avoid wasting time on pointless paperwork. Always deal with paperwork first thing in the day, and follow a general rule to deal with it once and once only. The two exceptions to this rule are matters that need to be addressed at a later date when more information becomes available, and documents that require serious reading in peace and quiet before you reply.

deal with it, **delegate** it or **destroy** it!

When you pick up an item, your response to it should be one of the following:

- dictate a reply
- pass it to a more appropriate person to deal with
- delegate it to your secretary
- delegate it to someone within your team
- throw it in the rubbish bin.

Telephone calls

Making telephone calls is another potential time-wasting activity. From experience, you have only a one in four chance of reaching the person you want to speak to. If possible, get someone else to make calls on your behalf and have them put calls through to you when the person you wish to speak to is on the line. Better still, use faxes or e-mail and ensure that incoming fax and e-mail messages are brought to your attention immediately.

Committees

It is always flattering to be asked to join a committee, but is your presence really needed? If not, politely decline the invitation. One of the first principles of efficiency is learning to say no – politely, indirectly perhaps, but firmly. If your timetable is busy, don't join another committee or add another regular commitment until you can drop something that you are already involved with.

Being assertive and staying in control

Learning to say 'no' is important, but being assertive is certainly not the same as being aggressive. To be assertive, you must be clear in your own mind what you want, be able to express your opinion clearly and be prepared to do so. You should always try to offer advice, information and solutions to problems rather than just complaining about them. Finally, if you do not understand something, be prepared to ask for clarification and advice or information from others when you need it. Inevitably, assertion and aggression interrelate when confronting someone behaving wrongly or inappropriately, but in almost every instance, this can, and should, be managed without aggression. Above all, always try to stay in control, not only of yourself, but also of the situation in hand.

Working as part of a team

Doctors can have some rather unfortunate characteristics. Younger ones tend to be aloof and arrogant, older ones cranky, and both tend to be rather paternalistic. Some can be verbally abusive and sarcastic in public and some even argue openly, which can be embarrassing and cruel to those on the receiving end. None of the above is an attractive trait. As a senior member of staff, you should set the standard of behaviour that everyone else follows.

Involve everyone in your decisions, be considerate to your co-workers and give credit when it is due. Remember that today's trainees are tomorrow's colleagues. Furthermore, to delegate effectively, you will need to have a good relationship with your team members – not one based on humiliation and abuse!

If you work in a group, as most of us do, always take into account the others in the group and the way in which they interact. The people you work with deserve your full confidence, and they should know that they have it. If someone interacts badly, within the group or with a patient, take that person aside and discuss the matter with him (with the aim of ensuring that the situation does not happen again). In this way, you can develop your team and your leadership of that team. Remember that your team is an extension of yourself and if an incident reflects badly on them, it also reflects badly on you.

Regardless of who you are dealing with, it is always best to say what you think tactfully, having thought the matter through thoroughly so that you are certain of your opinion. Some people are reluctant and embarrassed to say what they think, while others are inclined to say what the listener would like to hear, irrespective of what they really think. Ultimately, neither of these approaches is satisfactory. It is easiest and best to state a problem

be **honest** and **open** in your dealings with **colleagues**

clearly and give your view about its solution, whether you are advising a junior about his training or a consultant colleague about a clinical issue. This is also the key to effective mediation – identify the points of concern and then deal with them one by one, openly and honestly.

When the issue concerned is a matter of opinion rather than a matter of fact, things may be more complicated. However, the same principles still apply – identify the point for discussion and state your view clearly, however contentious. If the point for discussion is part of the agenda of a meeting and an immediate decision is going to be needed, it is sometimes a good idea to discuss the matter in advance with some of your colleagues. It is not always wise to make decisions on the spur of the moment, particularly if you are unsure of the views of the others involved in decision-making. A preliminary discussion will help make others aware of your point of view, and vice versa, so that any conflict of interest can be identified and discussed. It is then more likely that you will be able to persuade a group around to your way of thinking. At all times, avoid stating your views rudely or too forcefully, just speak directly – the difference between assertiveness and aggressiveness.

Effective clinical teams should, of course, put patients first. In particular, they should be able to demonstrate:

- purpose and value, including evidence of leadership, well-defined values, standards, functions and responsibilities, and strategic direction

- performance, including evidence of competent management, good systems, good performance records, effective internal performance monitoring, feedback and regular appraisal; in addition, all team members should accept responsibility for their own and each other's performance
- consistency, including evidence of thoroughness and a systematic approach to patient care
- effectiveness and efficiency, including evidence of thorough medical and clinical audit that the clinical team is continually assessing its care and outcomes
- a chain of responsibility, including evidence that the responsibilities of each of the team members are well defined and understood
- openness, such as a willingness for transparency to others, evidence of comparative external review and performance measures that can be easily understood by those outside the team
- overall acceptability, including evidence that the overall performance and results achieved by the team inspire the trust and confidence of patients, employers and professional colleagues.

Learning from criticism

An important component of success is learning to cope with both criticism and failure. No one is consistently successful. Indeed, Winston Churchill regarded success as "the ability to go from failure to failure without losing your enthusiasm".

In general, doctors do not take criticism well; however, failure obliges self-criticism and change. When used constructively, criticism can be instrumental in the search for future success. Doctors are currently subject to more criticism than ever before, as a result of societal changes and increased access to information. Patients no longer consider doctors to be omniscient and are not afraid to complain if things do not go according to plan.

Patients who complain about their care or treatment have a right to expect a prompt and appropriate response. As a doctor, you have a professional responsibility to deal with complaints constructively and honestly. You must also comply with any complaints procedure that applies to your work. Never allow a patient's complaint to prejudice the care or treatment you arrange for that individual.

Learning to accept criticism positively and live with your failures – patients who cannot be saved, research that does not reveal a significant result and so on – early on in your career will stand you in good stead for the future. Criticism is a gift; use the information provided constructively to make you a better doctor and person as a whole.

Being a good trainer

The most important aspect is to talk to your trainees and encourage them to respond honestly and openly without fear of recrimination. Most trainers are very busy doctors and training is yet another pressure on their time. It is very easy to allow a trainee to settle into a new job, and possibly a new hospital, and for you to be only vaguely aware of his performance except when he is actually in your presence. Your very 'busyness' may prevent him from talking to you because he doesn't wish to interrupt or appear rude. The trainee may leave, while you may have been only subconsciously aware that he was trying to approach you during his time with you. Positive action is required to prevent this from happening. Take time to greet a new trainee and arrange to meet when you have sufficient time – at least half an hour – to discuss adequately his past, the present attachment and his future. Set aside some time, about halfway through the attachment, to assess your trainee's progress, and then again to discuss his performance at the end of the attachment. Obviously, informal discussion during the attachment is valuable, but it is often impromptu and of ill-defined duration, so that matters cannot always be dealt with properly. The fact that time has formally been set aside does not mean that these discussions need to be formal, but they should be taken seriously. In addition, formal appraisals should be undertaken, as discussed previously; informal discussion and formal appraisal can be grouped together three times a year so long as sufficient time is allowed for both.

It is vital that you are aware of your trainee's needs, both overall and in relation to his particular stage of training. You should be aware of what is involved and able to answer questions about the organizational aspects of training, as well as helping with clinical development. If you do not answer his questions, who will? In any specialty that involves learning procedures, it is essential that these procedures are taught. It is easy to excuse doing something yourself rather than allowing your trainee to on the grounds that you yourself are able to do it more quickly and to a higher standard. Supervising your trainee may take longer and the procedure may not be done quite as well as you would like, but often the end result is just as satisfactory and is a far more beneficial experience for the trainee. Patience in such situations is not only a virtue, but also a necessity!

Further reading

Clay B. Flexible training – what are the opportunities? [career focus] *BMJ* 1998; 316(classified section 23 May):2–3.

Donald A. Effective teaching [career focus]. *BMJ* 1998;317(classified section 18 July):2–3.

Drife JO. Be interviewed. In: *How To Do It.* Vol 1, 2nd edn. London: *BMJ*, 1998.

Gatrell J, White A. *Medical Student to Medical Director, A Development Strategy for Doctors.* Bristol: NHS Training Division, 1995.

Gatrell J, White A. Appointing specialist registrars. *Clinician in Management* 1997;6.

Gatrell J, White A. Selecting doctors – making the most of the panel interview. Medical Interface. *J Dis Manage* 1997;February:21–3.

General Medical Council. *The New Doctor.* London: GMC, 1997.

Gray C. Time management [career focus]. *BMJ* 1998;316(classified section 4 April):2–3.

Hardern R. Starting a new consultant post [career focus]. *BMJ* 1998;317(classified section 17 October):2–3.

Harris D, Peyton R, Walker M. *Training the Trainers: Learning and Teaching.* Section 2 (Teaching in different situations). London: Royal College of Surgeons, 1996.

Quick TL. *Successful Team Building.* New York: Amacom, 1992.

The Department of Health. *The New NHS. Modern. Dependable. A National Framework for Assessing Performance.* London: DOH, 1998.

The Royal College of Surgeons. *Training the Trainers.* London: The Royal College of Surgeons of England, 1996.

Sharif K, Afnan M. Quality control in postgraduate training [career focus]. *BMJ* 1998;316(classified section 9 May):2–3.

making your name in private practice

"Never go to a doctor whose office plants have died"
Erma Bombeck in *Hammer and Tongues*

The freedom of patients to choose private practice and for doctors to work independently alongside the NHS is enshrined in the 1946 National Health Service Act. Unlike the NHS, where any improvement or development has to be laboriously agreed with committees, colleagues and managers, in private practice you can manage your own time, set your own agenda and create an independent working environment geared towards business-like efficiency and success.

Although one cannot discount the fact that private practice is likely to generate a satisfactory income, it also provides important opportunities for a doctor's personal and clinical development. Additional attractions include a pleasant working environment, more time to spend with each patient and the opportunity to investigate and deal with underlying problems rapidly and effectively.

The formative stages

From the time that you take up your consultant post, you are entitled to establish a private practice, provided that this does not interfere with your sessional commitments within the NHS. These will have been agreed at the time of your appointment, but can sometimes be renegotiated at a later date with the chief executive and medical director of your hospital.

Traditionally, doctors have been reluctant to discuss private practice and consequently this has made the business of setting up more difficult. In fact, the best approach is to be open and honest about your intentions, and discuss the issues with your colleagues. Although you may be concerned that they will resent the competition ('another mouth to feed'), you will find that most colleagues will wish you as much success in this arena as they do in your NHS role. They would not have appointed you initially if they did not think you worthy of success!

Ask your colleagues openly for advice about the best way to set up a private practice. Listen carefully to what they have to say, seek a second or even third opinion and then draw your own conclusions.

Getting started

There are a number of ways to get started in private practice. You can:

- take sessions in a private hospital
- start a private practice in your own home
- rent your own dedicated rooms.

Each of these initiatives has advantages and disadvantages.

Private hospital sessions

This is the cheapest and easiest option. This is usually a good way to start because you have the added advantage of working within a pleasant environment, with trained nursing staff and all the facilities you require for investigation of your patients. When you begin to work at a private hospital, they will often undertake a mailing on your behalf to inform referring GPs of your availability for consultations. In return, the hospital will usually charge you for the use of the facilities.

To get started, you should speak to the chief executive of your local private hospital and apply for admitting rights, which are usually granted by the medical advisory committee. The private hospital concerned will probably require references; your consultant colleagues may provide these, but it is always courteous to ask if they are willing to be referees, in the first instance.

Practising from home

Setting up in your own home is the time-honoured way to undertake private practice. Your home will need to be appropriate and the implications carefully considered in detail. You will also need to ensure that your consulting rooms are kept clean and tidy! Running a business from home can have tax implications and may render you liable to capital gains tax on your house. Before deciding on this option, you should discuss your plans in some detail with your accountant (see *Finance*, page 111).

Renting your own rooms

This is the most expensive option by far. However, it has the advantage that you will be available to see patients whenever you wish, and can have a secretary dedicated to taking calls and making appointments. Your own room becomes an extension of yourself. Personal effects, such as family photographs, in your office will provide your patients with visual clues about you. This insight will hopefully encourage patients to form a favourable opinion of you and make them feel more comfortable about choosing you as their doctor.

enter **private practice** with a **long-term strategic plan**

'Taking the plunge' in this way can be nail-biting stuff, but bear in mind that any new small business feels financially perilous for the first few months. Ultimately, long-term, strategic thinking, with an element of initial risk taking, is more likely to reap better rewards. However, it is possible to compromise by initially sharing rooms with a colleague – bearing in mind that many say one should choose one's consultant colleague more carefully than one's wife!

Staff

No man is an island and in private practice, just as in the NHS, a calm, efficient and effective team approach is needed. Your team is only as strong as its weakest link, and any problems should be addressed, not ignored.

Most importantly, appoint a dedicated, competent secretary. The telephone needs to be manned for referrals from 9 am to 5 pm, and your secretary should be personable, intelligent and 'on the ball'. Aim to employ someone with a positive attitude, and provide orientation and ongoing training. Strive to demonstrate the qualities that you expect of your secretary yourself. Avoid, for example, rolling your eyes to the ceiling when dealing with a difficult patient, or criticizing demanding relatives to your secretary. Although some people seem to enjoy it, negativity is rather contagious. It can permeate relationships with patients and staff alike and may impair the overall performance of your practice. Some people fall into this pattern without realizing it. It helps to imagine creating a chart for yourself and checking how many positive and negative statements you make in 1 hour. How would *you* like to have yourself as a doctor, boss, spouse or friend?

Although your secretary is your most important team member (and one who has the power to make or break your practice), other team members each have an essential part to play.

- Is the receptionist welcoming and polite?
- If investigations are needed, are they completed in a well-organized, dignified and efficient manner?
- Are the results always accessible?
- If a patient needs to be admitted, are the hospital staff cheerful, friendly and competent, and aware of the reason for admission?
- Finally, if the patient leaves a message with your secretary, do you always reply promptly, effectively and professionally?

Working with colleagues

A weakness of private practice is the tendency for doctors to work alone. In fact, as in the NHS, teamwork is vital. If you are a surgeon, your key partner is your anaesthetist and it is important that you both work in harmony. For example, do you both provide the same information to patients? Do you both provide adequate pre- and postoperative patient review? Also, his fee schedule should be compatible with yours.

Arranging cover

Another important consideration is the provision of medical cover when you are unavailable. Many private hospitals are introducing on-call rotas for consultants to ensure that there is always a consultant available to deal with unexpected emergencies. Remember, you must be satisfied that, when you are off duty, suitable arrangements are made to cover your own patients' medical care. These arrangements should include effective hand-over procedures and clear communication, ideally written, between the doctors concerned. Be sure that the individual who is standing in for you has the experience, knowledge and skills to deal with the cases for which he will be responsible.

There is a growing trend for private practitioners to work in groups. For example, four orthopaedic surgeons, experienced in different areas, might practice on a rota basis, referring patients on within the team to the appropriate expert. This type of private group practice is likely to become more prevalent in the future.

Marketing your practice

In the UK, most patients gain access to a specialist via their GP. Therefore, marketing your practice largely depends on making referring physicians aware of your presence. In marketing, it is accepted that the average business never hears from 96% of its happy customers. However, an unhappy customer voices his concerns to, on average,

> remember, an **unhappy customer voices** his **concerns widely**

nine or ten people – among them, in your case, undoubtedly the referring GP! Customers whose complaints are resolved tell, on average, only five people, and some of what they say may be positive.

You should be able to offer expertise and technology that will allow you to diagnose and resolve the problems of the GP's patients speedily and accurately. Other factors influencing whether patients are referred to you or to someone else include ease and speed of access to you, efficiency of feedback and whether or not patients are satisfied with their overall management and outcome.

Interaction with GPs can be achieved in a number of ways. Doctors starting out in private practice can send a mailing to all GPs in the area. If you move premises subsequently, another mailing is appropriate. Rules concerning advertising have recently been relaxed by the GMC, but it is still wise to be cautious about direct marketing to referring doctors. It is certainly inappropriate to criticize or denigrate a colleague or to claim that you offer a better service than a competitor, but a statement about your specific expertise, availability and how you can be contacted is acceptable, provided that it is factual and verifiable. In most parts of the UK, GPs will not refer private patients to you unless you and your team deliver a good service to their NHS patients.

Regular contact with your referral sources is invaluable. Articles you may write for journals read extensively by GPs, such as the *BMJ* and *Pulse*, are indirect but valuable methods of marketing yourself and enhancing your reputation. Presentations to GPs in postgraduate centres, where direct contact with your referring doctor can also be made in workshops and during the pre- or post-meeting meal, are similarly useful. You may also meet GPs at social events.

Direct marketing to patients is less important in the UK than in the USA because, in the UK, most patients are referred by their GPs and insurance companies are often reluctant to pay for those who are not. However, brochures for your patients with information about your practice are valuable. They should include the advice that patients cannot usually be seen without a referral from a GP. They should be well written and designed, as well as informative, presenting a little information about you and a list of charges that the patient can expect. Although many doctors are reluctant to be up-front about their charges, patients almost always prefer them to be, as it allows them to clarify the extent of their cover with their insurer and relieves them of uncertainty about their liability. Approximately 20% of all private patients are uninsured and cover their own costs. A fixed-price package eases concern about unlimited liability for such patients. Brochures can be pre-tested on your patients before the final version is produced. Ask questions such as 'If you could change one thing about this pamphlet, what would it be?'

Another way to improve your practice is to conduct patient surveys after treatment, assessing every stage in the service delivery. Assess satisfaction at each point of patient contact:
- original phone calls
- first consultation
- investigations

- treatment visits
- follow-up queries.

Ask, for example, 'How important is X to your overall satisfaction? And how well did we meet your expectations at Y?' Ensure that this exercise is meaningful – be prepared to act on the results of your survey.

Dealing with private patients

Success in private practice relies not only on referral from GPs, but also on recommendations from other patients. The quality of service that you offer is critical if word is to get around that you are *the* person to see for a certain problem. Of course, as with NHS patients, the following important principles apply:

- listen to patients and respect their views
- always treat patients professionally and considerately
- respect patients' privacy and dignity
- treat information about patients as confidential
- give patients the advice they ask for or need about their condition, its treatment and prognosis.

> the **quality** of **service you offer** is **critical**

Put yourself in the position of a patient who is worried about a symptom or condition and decides to call your practice to make an appointment.

- How many times does the telephone ring before it is answered?
- How polite and efficient is your secretary?
- What is the earliest appointment you can offer?

When the patient walks into your office, he will make a rapid value judgement about whether he feels confident to have you as his doctor. Although this judgement will be made on much the same basis as that made by a NHS patient, he will be very aware that he is paying for the consultation, and thus may have higher expectations.

A number of factors will influence how comfortable the patient feels about you:

- your reputation as a caring and successful doctor, which goes before you and strongly influences patients' opinions

- the way you communicate to the patient that you care about his problem, and that you have the expertise to diagnose and treat it
- your physical environment, as patients will inevitably judge you by the setting they find you in
- your expertise in managing his problem.

With regard to your reputation, this is acquired only by the cumulative impact of a series of satisfied patients and good outcomes. For this, and other reasons, it is critical that you do not over-extend yourself in private practice. One serious complication and its consequences can undo years of good results. In medicine, unnecessary risk-taking is hazardous and best avoided!

Using the latest technology

Private practice lends itself rather well to the use of the latest office technology. A number of user-friendly patient database systems are available. With the advent of scanners, it is possible to run a near-paperless office, creating a 'high-tech' image that is generally appreciated by patients. It is essential that each and every result or letter is scanned in as soon as it arrives; methodical and efficient backing up of files is mandatory. It is necessary, however, to retain a paper record for medicolegal purposes for at least 10 years. If your patients' files are wholly on computer, keeping paper records in chronological day files rather than in duplicate patient files will save hours of laborious sorting. Although a computer on your desk may convey the correct image, beware of being glued to your screen, and thereby losing eye and personal contact with your patient.

keeping **accurate records** is **essential**

Developing your own website is the next frontier in the marketing of private practice. In the USA, many doctors have these and it will not be long before they are common in the UK. As with your brochure, this should be written in easy-to-read, plain English, and should set out the nature of your expertise. Some background information on the main conditions that you treat can be helpful, but these are often best supplied via links to larger, reputable, often US-based websites.

Using new technologies in the treatment of your patients can also be a way of boosting private practice. Minimally invasive devices, such as lasers, have a tremendous appeal to patients and are often marketed on your behalf by the manufacturer and installed in private hospitals at their expense. Unfortunately, the results gained using these devices do not always live up to the initial hype. Moreover, your long-term credibility depends on you backing winners, so beware of espousing too avidly a new method that later turns out to be a dead donkey!

Dealing with insurance companies

Health insurers can be like any other insurer – some seem to offer comprehensive cover until you make a claim, when you may find that the small print precludes that particular eventuality! Helping your patients through the maze of procedures involved in health insurance is an integral part of private practice.

When discussing health insurance with a patient, you must make it clear that he enters into a contract with you. Strictly speaking, the issue of whether the patient's insurance company will cover the cost of your fees is between the patient and his insurer. He should call the company's helpdesk to check that his consultations and in-patient procedures are covered. In practice, if you want to be reimbursed for your time and effort, you or a member of your team will need to facilitate the process of dealing with the insurance company.

Most private insurers will reimburse only for acute rather than chronic illness. Many will require a claim form to be completed, on which the date of onset of the condition and the date of referral are usually requested. Learn to use the OPCS procedure codes to classify diagnosis and treatment. Many companies also ask for the estimated waiting time for an NHS consultation for the patient's condition.

Avoiding pitfalls

Never stray outside your specialist area, however tempting it is to help out the patient by doing so. If problems occur, you must have the skills to deal with them. If you are dabbling in another specialty, this expertise will probably be lacking.

A second potential pitfall lies in the way in which you deal with complaints or complications that fall within your disease area. Be apologetic, honest and straightforward with patients and take the time to explain exactly what the problem is, what the short- and long-term problems are and what you intend to do about it. If a second opinion is needed, arrange for a senior colleague or a senior specialist in the relevant area to see the patient.

never stray from your **area** of **expertise**

Document all stages of the process clearly and accurately, and keep all parties fully informed. You should not withhold any relevant information. Do not be afraid to contact your medical defence union for advice – this is what you are paying for. If complications do occur, exercise sensitivity when submitting your bill. Receipt of an invoice after a long and protracted illness can be the final straw that persuades an unhappy patient to contact his solicitor!

In some specialties, such as dermatology, and obstetrics and gynaecology, it may be appropriate to perform minor procedures in your rooms rather than in the operating theatre. If you do so, remember that the same strict rules that are enforced in the NHS regarding sterility and the disposal of human waste and sharp objects, such as needles and scalpels, are applicable to private practice and must be adhered to scrupulously.

Remember, in private practice, as in NHS medicine, you must not:

- use your position to establish improper personal relationships with patients or their close relatives
- improperly disclose or misuse confidential information about patients
- give, or recommend, to patients an investigation or treatment that you know is not in their best interest
- enable anyone who is not registered with the GMC to carry out tasks that require the training, knowledge and skills of a doctor – for example, to assist you in theatre.

Don't forget though that when you get it right private practice can be immensely satisfying and produce the highest standard of patient care.

effective communication

"I ask only for information"
Rosa Dartle in *David Copperfield*

Clear, concise and effective communication is essential in all aspects of medicine. To be a more successful doctor, you must develop the ability to establish a rapid rapport, first and foremost with patients, but also with colleagues, managers and other healthcare professionals. Good communication depends not only on content but also on delivery. Both need to be adjusted according to the audience and the setting in which you find yourself.

Talking to your patients

Talking to patients is not always easy, particularly in the setting of the busy clinic or the wards. There are, however, a number of golden rules that, if followed, will help you to do this effectively.

As a patient enters your office or cubicle, stand up and shake his hand. Make a 'connection' by listening attentively and avoid interrupting – one study suggested that most doctors interrupt within 19 seconds of the interview commencing! Establish eye contact and always try to be concerned, interested and focused. Ensure that you allow yourself sufficient time to glean all the salient points of the case and, when appropriate, perform a gentle and professional physical examination. You should give your opinion emphatically, but in a friendly and sympathetic way. Throughout the consultation, take care to speak clearly and concisely, avoiding medical jargon, acronyms and technical terms. Listen *to* your patient, don't talk *at* him.

When it comes to treatment, discuss the pros and cons of each option with your patient. Listen to your patient's opinions; he is more likely to comply with a treatment plan into which he has had some input. Nowadays, the concept of a doctor–patient partnership has replaced the paternalism of old. Important messages still need to be repeated and reinforced several times because stressed and anxious patients may absorb only a fraction of what they are told. It may be helpful for the patient if you write down the key points or draw a quick sketch for them to take away.

Never give the impression that you are in a hurry. Be sure to switch off your mobile phone and avoid having phone calls put through to you during a consultation. You do not want your patient to think someone else's time is more important to you than theirs.

Remain focused on the case throughout the consultation; at the end, summarize the agreed treatment plan, stand up and escort your patient to the door and shake hands again, maintaining eye contact. Make sure that the follow-up arrangements are understood. If possible, give your patient literature that provides relevant and understandable information about his condition. Tell patients about support groups and make contact details available. Make it clear that you care.

The Internet: breakthrough or breakdown?

There can be no doubt that the Internet is responsible for a huge information explosion. Patients now have access to more information regarding their conditions and treatments than ever before, although much of it is unregulated and seldom evidence-based. We have all been confronted with patients bearing reams and reams of Internet print-outs! It is likely that much of this material has been generated outside the European Union, and the legislation that governs it is very different from that in the UK. For example, in the USA prescription-only medicines can be promoted directly to patients, while this is illegal within the European Union.

patients have access to more information than ever before

When prescribed a new treatment or particularly when newly diagnosed with a disease, many patients crave information. Unfortunately, much information found on the Internet is for marketing purposes and can often be unreliable. Knowledge that the patient has gained from less authoritative sources may be used to challenge your position and undermine the doctor–patient relationship, which will take time and patience to re-establish.

The Internet is a powerful tool for change that is already proving invaluable. However, it is unlikely that complete control will ever be achieved, and only an integrated approach between patients, healthcare professionals, governments and pharmaceutical companies will limit the potential problems. There is no question that the Internet is set to change all of our lives, and we must not get left behind.

Breaking bad news

How bad news should be conveyed to patients and relatives is seldom taught or even discussed by doctors. As malignancies and other potentially fatal conditions are commonplace, you may find yourself in the position of delivering bad news. For a patient, to be told that he or she is suffering from a terminal illness is a defining moment that will never be forgotten. Historically, doctors have shied away from telling their patients the truth: in 1672, the French physician Samuel de Sobière considered the idea, but discounted it on the grounds that it might seriously jeopardize his medical practice!

In 1961, a landmark paper by Oken revealed that 90% of surgeons in the USA would not routinely discuss a diagnosis of cancer with their patients. Subsequent studies, however, showed that a growing number of patients wanted to know about and understand their diagnosis. Attitudes in this respect have adapted gradually, particularly in the USA, such that a repeat survey, almost 20 years after the original, showed that US physicians had completely reversed their attitudes, with more than 90% saying they would tell a patient if they had cancer. This change has not necessarily been mirrored in other parts of the world: in the UK, a survey of family physicians and hospital consultants in the early 1980s showed that 75% and 56%, respectively, did not routinely tell their patients the truth about a cancer diagnosis.

It is not difficult to understand the main reasons why clinicians wish to avoid sharing bad news with their patients. It can be a harrowing experience to be the harbinger of doom, and subsequently have to provide patients with the support they need while they absorb and grapple with the nature of their illness. Traditionally, clinicians have found two main justifications for keeping patients in the dark. First, the facts may upset them. This is undoubtedly the case, but this line of reasoning is not acceptable to any other profession in which news may be bad, for example, stockbrokers or lawyers. Second, doctors, and sometimes close relatives, presume that patients do not really want to know.

In fact, several studies have confirmed the opposite to be true. In a survey of 250 patients attending a cancer centre in Scotland, 79% wanted to know as much as possible about their disease and 96% specifically wanted to know if their disease was cancer. Almost all patients wanted to know their realistic chance of cure and to be given details about possible side-effects of treatment. They also wanted to decide who else should be told. All patients felt that family members should be informed provided that the patient had given permission, but nearly two-thirds felt that if the patient did not wish relatives to know, then the family should not be taken into confidence.

Sharing with your patient

How, then, should a caring physician break bad news to a patient newly diagnosed as suffering from a life-threatening condition? Not surprisingly, most doctors feel uneasy when in such a position and perhaps anxiety about communication techniques underlies most arguments for not telling the patient the truth. Many of us have had little or no counselling training, and are often pushed for time in our busy clinics. The difficulty is to convey the information sensitively and supportively, and in a way that the patient can understand. You should not appear rushed. Many of our own patients have admitted that they understood hardly anything

provide **written information** that can be **referred** to **later**

they were told in the traumatic interview when the bad news was broken: "As soon as you said the word *cancer*, doctor, my mind went blank." Try to find a quiet, private place, where interruptions are unlikely, to convey the news. Also, attempt to develop a connection with the patient and then offer to share the news with him rather than simply blurting it out. It is important to counterbalance bad news with support and information.

Having a close relative in the consulting room means there is a second person to absorb the information, as well as to provide emotional support to the affected individual. Providing written information about the disease, which can be digested later when the patient has recovered from the initial impact of the news, is usually much appreciated. Easy-to-understand literature should be available, as patients often have a large number of questions. Ideally, specially trained nurses should be at hand to provide counselling and support for patients, both immediately upon disclosure of the diagnosis of a terminal illness and afterwards as the news gradually sinks in. Information on specific patient-support groups can also be very helpful – many now have a presence on the Internet.

Supporting close relatives

The impact of cancer on a patient's partner is another important, but often neglected, area of concern. For example, the treatments used in prostate cancer commonly affect sexual function and these need to be discussed not only with the patient, but also with his spouse. The consequences of loss of libido, erectile dysfunction and ejaculatory disturbances must be explained sympathetically to both partners. Failure to do so effectively may have a devastatingly negative impact on their relationship. Men, and older men in particular, diagnosed as suffering from cancer are particularly reliant on the social support that stems from intimate relationships, and withdrawal from sexual relationships may have severe consequences on both their quality of life and overall health. Sympathetic, unhurried counselling of the couple about this aspect of their lives, as well as about treatment and its possible side-effects, is vital.

The essential skills

Learning how to break bad news sympathetically and effectively is an essential skill to acquire. Nowadays, there is no excuse for the clinician who simply does not want to perform this important part of his job. It is an essential part of a doctor's role and, with attention to detail, can be done well. Aptly, it has been said that, "If the breaking of bad news is done badly, patients and their families may never forgive us; in contrast, if we get it right they will never forget us." The challenge for clinicians everywhere is to improve this important aspect of their communication skills.

Communicating with dying patients

Death doesn't always come to us as a friend, and in no other situation is good communication between doctors, patient and relatives more important, or potentially more fraught. Remember that, in a family, death is associated with all sorts of concomitant tensions. Not only are the relatives trying to deal with the demise of a loved one, but they may also be having to confront other compromising issues, such as financial hardship, feelings of guilt and problematic family relationships.

One problem of which we should be acutely aware is the lack of public understanding about the way today's NHS functions. Many people have fond memories of how things were years ago - matrons, plenty of beds and access to the same doctor continually. However, things have changed. The level of emergency admissions means that patients are placed where a bed is available, often on wards nursed by staff not familiar with a particular patient's condition. This inevitably leads to fragmented communication. In addition, the reduction in junior doctors' hours makes it less likely that a familiar doctor will be available to talk to relatives. Attitudes of the public have also changed. The assumption that the doctor is necessarily right has been undermined and there is a much greater reluctance to accept death as an inevitable outcome, no matter how old or how ill the patient.

The key to the problem is good communication. Lack of information makes people feel powerless, and powerlessness can lead to aggression. Doctors need to communicate effectively with all members of the medical team. Timely and appropriate information must be given to the patient and relatives in a friendly, professional and sympathetic manner. In the words of Dame Cicely Saunders, founder of the hospice movement, "Remember, five minutes conversation on a timely basis can save hours of work later on. It is not so much the *quantity* of time, but the *quality* of time that is critical."

Communicating with colleagues and managers

To be 'successful' as a doctor, you have to be perceived as such by your colleagues and managers – this is your 'reputation'. The way in which you communicate with them on clinical or academic matters is critical to the position in which they place you in their own mental hierarchy. It may

Effective communication

seem blindingly obvious, but keep in mind that people prefer a friendly, affable, optimistic colleague to a taciturn, abrasive and pessimistic one, and are far more likely to relate to and support the former.

As doctors meet so many colleagues, first impressions are particularly important. Shaking hands, maintaining eye contact and remembering the name of a new acquaintance is helpful. Sir Yehudi Menuhin, arguably the most successful musician of the 20th century, used to visit his music school only once or twice a year, but would always make an effort to speak to each and every pupil, and remember their names and details.

> your **reputation**
> **depends** on your
> **interactions** with others

Coping with the media

Dealing with the media is an increasingly important communication skill for the modern doctor and an excellent way of raising your own profile. The best way to acquire this is to attend a media skills course, at which you will be able to obtain some practical experience through radio and television interview role play and subsequent post-mortem audiovisual analysis of your performance.

When dealing with the media, at all times think of the image you are trying to create – caring, composed and competent – and the one you are trying to avoid, that of being aloof, arrogant and defensive. On television, body language is critical in this respect. Remember to look directly at the interviewer or camera. Try to look relaxed. Avoid adopting defensive body positions and fiddling with your hands, nose or ears. Use gestures sparingly. Even raising a finger during a television interview can look like an exaggerated and aggressive gesture to the viewers. In radio interviews, keep your audience and message in mind at all times. Speak slowly and clearly, and avoid using medical jargon. To give yourself time to think, rephrase the question as the start to your answer. Avoid beginning with 'er...'.

Remember that your best weapon is your clinical skill and experience. TV and radio journalists seldom attack doctors, although this is changing in the current climate. If you are criticized, respond positively – try to convey the message that medicine is not an easy business but in spite of this the vast majority of cases go well. Keep your answers simple, short and straightforward. Before the interview, try to think of a catchy 'sound-bite' that encapsulates your message, and end the interview on an upbeat and positive note.

Caution is needed when dealing with newspaper or magazine journalists. Beware making an impromptu remark that may be taken out of context and splashed across the front page. Remember that medicine is full of 'human-interest' stories that the newspapers love. Above all, avoid breaching patient confidentiality or denigrating your colleagues publicly. Before accepting a call from a journalist, think carefully about what you want to say and try to put a positive spin on the issue in question. For example, you might point out that although one wrong kidney was removed recently at St Elsewhere's, some 7999 successful operations were performed in the same year.

Making oral presentations

Good presentations do not just happen – they are the result of careful planning and preparation. Interesting and relevant content, clear delivery and a variety of visual and auditory techniques all contribute to an effective presentation. To paraphrase Tolstoy's opening line of *Anna Karenina*: "Good presentations are all alike; every bad presentation is bad in its own way."

Developing the text

The spoken word needs to be much simpler and more straightforward than the written word. To make your message clear, remember the adage: "Tell them what you are going to tell them, tell them, and then tell them what you have told them." Use plain, simple English and try to illustrate your points with word pictures; many people will remember information that is told as a story or anecdote rather than dry facts or ideas.

Know your audience. Avoid the 'So what?' factor by asking yourself "What is the audience hoping to get out of this talk?" At the same time, consider your message and how best to convey it. Make it clear very early on in the talk why your subject is relevant and exactly 'what's in it' for the attendees. Be clear about what you want the audience to take away with them. Also consider the setting – find out who or what will precede and follow your talk. Make sure that your presentation fits in with the general theme.

It is crucial to be thoroughly prepared for your presentation:

- research your topic and write one long draft – set out all your ideas and facts
- work through this draft and underline the key points
- write these out on separate pieces of paper, and then go back to your first draft and find statements, facts or examples that corroborate your main points – use these sparingly
- your audience's time is precious – do not waste it with inappropriate or irrelevant information
- use logical development and try to link one major point with the next
- mark the points that can be made more effectively with a slide or overhead.

Preparing your delivery

However well prepared your text, it will not be appreciated unless it is well delivered in a lively, enthusiastic fashion. Do not memorize your talk – you risk forgetting a segment and grinding to an embarrassing and seemingly eternal halt. If this happens at a major presentation, believe me, you will blush at the memory for a very long time! Write the key points on numbered cards. You will also have your slides or overheads as prompts, but avoid using them as a crutch by following them slavishly. Practise your talk four or five times. Do not just run through it silently – actually try to recreate the setting and speak your words out loud. Check the facilities, such as slide-changing buttons, carefully before you ascend the podium!

always **deliver enthusiastically**

Delivery

After your talk, people will leave not only with the information that you have supplied (if they have listened), but also with an impression of you.

This stems not from what you say, but how you say it. Body language is an important part of your image.

- Try to stand squarely towards the audience, with legs slightly apart.
- Use appropriate hand gestures to emphasize your words and establish eye contact with your audience.
- Do not talk to your slides – you will inevitably turn away from the audience and the microphone.
- Do not overuse the laser pointer, particularly if nerves produce a hand tremor!
- Dress comfortably and appropriately – if most of the attendees are wearing suits, then you should be wearing one, and if most are casually dressed, you should be smart but casual too.

Avoid the monotonous delivery that sedates an audience so effectively! Smile and enthuse – if you are not interested in your subject, why should your audience be? Use voice inflection, pauses, tone and pace – speak slowly, loudly and deliberately. Humour is a powerful way to establish and maintain audience rapport. But making people laugh is not a matter of telling jokes. In general, avoid jokes unless you can deliver them with timing and congruence – a joke that falls flat stays down a long time, along with your talk! 'Fun' is not the same as 'funny'; often all you need to do to raise a smile and get the audience on your side is point out the odd or unusual aspects of something quite mundane.

Visual aids

Good slides or overheads will add interest to your presentation and provide another medium for communicating your key messages. They allow an audience to focus on the salient points. However, unclear, cluttered slides with spelling mistakes will do little to enhance your image and credibility. Follow the golden rules for effective visuals (Table 4).

Always check the size of the room that you will be presenting in. Ensure that people at the back of the room will be able to read your slides, otherwise you risk losing their attention. Do not try to present too many slides – allow each slide to be shown long enough for everyone to read. As a guideline, a 15-minute presentation should be accompanied by no more than 15 slides.

Effective communication

Table 4

Making the most of slides and overheads

- Each slide or overhead should have a specific purpose. Limit each to one main idea
- Be accurate – mistakes on visuals stand out like a sore thumb, forcing the speaker into an apologetic mode
- Aim for simplicity and conciseness – do not overload your slide with information
- Design slides so that the back row of your audience can see and understand them. If your slide is readable without any magnification when held up to a light, it should be effective when projected
- Use strong, bold sans serif typefaces. Don't use all capitals – lower case letters are more legible
- Use ample spacing between lines, no more than seven words per line and a maximum of seven lines per slide
- Ensure axes and data lines on graphs are sufficiently bold to be clearly visible
- Avoid punctuation; use bullet points
- Use light-coloured text (ideally yellow or white) on a dark background
- Use a consistent style between slides – slides can then be mixed and matched for future presentations
- Summarize the 'take-home' messages on your final slide

Using PowerPoint™ presentations

Increasing numbers of people are using Microsoft PowerPoint™ software to make presentations directly from their own laptop or a computer disk. These can be very effective and do project an image of someone who is forward thinking and able to work with the latest technology. There are some pitfalls, however, because of the potential glitches associated with using any computer. Take time to learn how to use the software properly – there are many short courses and good manuals available.

Immediately before your presentation, ensure that your computer and projector are working properly. There is nothing worse than standing on the podium looking abject because your slides do not appear on the screen. Avoid cluttering your slides and including information that draws attention away from yourself. Do not overuse the 'animation' that PowerPoint allows – remember that in good communication less is more!

Handling questions

Question time can be nerve-racking, but it can also be fun and the highlight of your talk! Responding naturally and effectively to the audience is the best way to get them on your side. Try to avoid answering too quickly, or giving too detailed an answer. Repeat the question and then answer clearly and briefly. Do not let one questioner – particularly a dominant and aggressive one – monopolize your time. Instead, move on to another, hopefully more positive, questioner. You can do this by pointing out that only one question is allowed from any member of the audience and turning away to a different part of the auditorium, although strictly speaking this is the chairman's responsibility. Use question time as an opportunity to repeat your message. Always end on a positive, 'high' note – many good presentations are spoilt by a lack of confidence when closing. Try not to rush from the podium, obviously relieved to have survived your ordeal! Remove your lapel microphone, smile and return to your seat in the auditorium in a cool and composed manner.

Poster presentations

As the number of people attending international conferences continues to grow, posters are being used increasingly as a method of communicating research data to a wide audience. Posters are a very effective and flexible tool, allowing viewers to study information in as much or as little detail as they wish. Good preparation is essential – read any instructions carefully and adhere to them. Do not try to overload the poster with information. Ensure that the text is concise, simple and supported with appropriate graphics. Divide the content into the following sections:

- aims
- introduction
- methods

- results
- conclusions
- references.

Carefully consider the design aspects of the poster. Make sure the text is large enough to be read at a short distance, and do not introduce too many different fonts as this will detract from the content. Use colour judiciously and sparingly, considering the overall visual impact of the poster, while trying to make it both attractive and informative. If you have to present your poster, do so without slides, summarizing the key points of the work succinctly – it is not an opportunity to give a 7-minute lecture! Always be enthusiastic, confident and professional.

Chairing small meetings and committees

The way in which you chair committees or meetings can greatly influence your peers' and colleagues' perception of you. By being prepared, you will develop a reputation for being a reliable chairman. Your role as chairman of a meeting is to manage:
- individual speakers
- the group
- yourself.

To do this effectively requires thorough planning; too many chairmen arrive at the last moment and try to 'wing it'. This is a great time-waster and is discourteous to all in attendance. Ideally, you should have studied and thought about the session in some detail, prepared relevant questions and, if possible, made arrangements to meet each of the speakers or participants prior to the session. By taking the following actions, you will ensure that every attendee gets the most from the meeting and that the meeting fulfils its objectives:

thorough planning ensures **successful chairmanship**

- circulate the agenda and talk to colleagues before the meeting; if possible, establish whether they are potential supporters or opposers of the scheme(s) you have in mind

- arrive early and start on time, make the necessary introductions, run through the agenda, but allow everybody to have their say
- be pleasant, but firm and direct; never show irritability, argue or make personal remarks about individuals – people tend not to forget them and may harbour a grudge for years afterwards
- always try to finish punctually, making a succinct and upbeat summary of the session. Thank each of the speakers and members of the group for their participation.

Chairing academic sessions

The success of an academic session depends not only on the quality of the science presented, but also on the way in which information is delivered. Consequently, being asked to chair an academic session should be considered a privilege, and is a role not to be undertaken lightly. As chairman, you will need to manage the session carefully. Therefore, you must set the guidelines for the session, facilitate the discussion and summarize the take-home messages in a simple, concise and relevant way.

Prior to the meeting, you should:
- meet the speakers, stressing the importance of keeping to the allocated time and leaving sufficient time for questions
- agree a timing signal, and agree a procedure should the presentation over-run
- decide how questions will be handled
- agree a signal the speaker should use should he want the chairman to intervene.

Remember, you never have a second chance to make a first impression, and what you wear is fundamental to this. Dressing too casually will suggest that the meeting is not important, whereas smart clothing will project the correct image. You should also appear confident and professional, but remain calm and relaxed throughout the proceedings.

Establishing eye contact with both the speaker and audience will convey your interest and involvement in the session. When each talk is over, make eye contact with the speaker to put him at ease. Be careful not to display any form of body language that communicates a lack of interest to the audience – never fidget and look bored!

Effective communication

Opening the session

Your objectives at the start of a session are to generate interest among and engage the attention of the audience, encouraging them to be receptive to the presentations. By introducing yourself and briefly mentioning your credentials for the job, you will begin to establish a rapport with the audience. Highlight the objective of the session and enthuse the audience by stating its relevance to them: describe how the session will be structured and how questions will be handled.

Handling questions effectively

Managing the questions session is perhaps one of the biggest challenges of chairmanship. Clearly, it is the responsibility of the speakers to respond to the questions, but as chairman, you too should play an active role. When a talk finishes, thank the speaker and encourage the audience to provide their perspective. Calculate in advance how much time to allow for each question, and keep the discussion flowing to allow as many people as possible to participate. Make sure each questioner states their name and institution before asking his question. You should always have a question or two prepared in case there are none from the floor.

Although most are fairly straightforward, there are occasions when peripheral questions or rambling questioners may serve to distract from the objective of the session. Take control of the situation, perhaps suggesting that the questioner meet with the speaker after the session. Ensure that dominant personalities do not monopolize the proceedings, and that those with the most to contribute have an opportunity to do so. When all the questions have been asked or time has run out, do not let the session peter out – close it on a positive note.

Publications

Before committing yourself to any writing or editing project, find out about the expected publication schedule. Proceed with the project only if you are confident that you will be able to give it the attention that it deserves throughout the duration of its production. There is nothing more frustrating for a publisher or editor than an author who does not deliver or needs to be repeatedly chased. This will not win you friends or respect, and if word spreads that you are a 'non-deliverer', invitations to contribute to publications in the future will not be forthcoming.

Writing

Writing is a skill, not a talent, and can be improved by practice and careful thought. Clarity is your goal and this can be achieved with careful planning and meticulous attention to detail. Although you may feel that there is a world of difference between writing an article for a peer-reviewed journal and perhaps becoming involved with writing for patients, the basic principles are the same (Table 5).

The most vital questions to ask yourself are 'Who is my reader?' and 'What is my message?' Keep these in mind throughout the writing process.

Now, what is your brief? Are you writing a paper for submission to a journal, a poster or a chapter for a book, perhaps? Look at the guidelines carefully and, if possible, look at some samples of the type of work wanted. Do you really need an introduction? How detailed does the discussion of your methods need to be? Should you include figures and tables, and if so, in what format? And what level of referencing is required? At all costs, avoid thinking that you know what is wanted without double-checking. One of the age-old problems that editors encounter is finding that authors have written what they want to write, rather than what they have actually been asked for.

The next step is to research the topic, and then put all your ideas, supporting facts and arguments down on paper. Start by drafting an outline. From there, it is not too difficult to organize your main points in order of importance, adding details to support each main point. At this stage, you are ready to write. Stick to the outline and start with the main ideas and their supporting details. Once this is done, revise the text and consider how well your message has been conveyed.

writing is a **skill**, not a **talent**

Effective communication

Table 5

Effective writing

- Avoid trying to impress the reader with your expansive vocabulary. If you find yourself reaching for a thesaurus, put it down immediately!
- Try to use as few words as possible – most of what we write is far too verbose. Think in terms of having to pay for lineage, as you would if you were writing an advertisement. However, do not slip into note-like prose
- Use short words rather than long ones
- Use jargon and acronyms only when writing exclusively for fellow specialists
- Restrict sentences to 15–20 words. Aim to introduce only one 'idea' per sentence or clause
- Use your words with accuracy. For example, if you wrote the phrase 'around 15–20 words', 'around' is redundant as the range automatically implies 'around' to the reader
- Use bullet points to avoid hiding lengthy lists in your text (they help to break up text and make it less visually daunting)
- Use different levels of headings (having checked the style of the publication, of course). These also help to break up the text
- Avoid clichés like the plague(!)
- Make sure that arithmetic is correct and that any statistics are accurate
- Keep your reader and your message in mind at all times

Submitting to a journal

If you are submitting a paper to a peer-reviewed journal, you will have to deal with reviewers' comments and will probably be expected to check page proofs (see page 75). If, for some reason, you find that you will not have the opportunity to check your submitted article before publication, scrutinize it closely before submission – pay particular attention to drug regimens and dosages, experimental data and the results of any calculations. Also, double-check the results of any other studies that you may have included in your introduction or discussion. Follow the instructions for submission of articles carefully and always keep copies of everything that you send to the journal.

Working with a medical communications or public relations agency

Writing for a pharmaceutical company-sponsored publication can be both lucrative and satisfying – publications are usually of the highest quality and it can be a thrill to see your name adorning such a good piece of work. However, your first encounter with this type of company may be something of a shock. You may be approached by either a product manager or other representative from a pharmaceutical company, or by an account manager or editor of the agency working on the pharmaceutical company's behalf. Before committing yourself to anything, you must make sure that you are completely clear about your role, the aim of the publication, how your name will be used, who has editorial control, how much work is involved and the schedule.

The type of project varies widely, but each and every publication has a role in marketing the company's drug or product. You may simply be asked to write a short article on your specialist subject, which will be very lightly edited, returned to you for approval and then published. Fine. Will the pharmaceutical company's logo be flashed across the cover? Very likely. If you are not

> before **accepting** an **invitation** be **clear** about **your role**

happy with such an association, then steer well clear of this type of work.

At the other end of the scale, you may be asked to put your name to a piece of work that has been drafted on your behalf. Be cautious about this – agree only if it reflects accurately your own convictions. This approach may seem favourable in terms of efficiency of time, but this is not always the case. Although you will save time at the outset, you must invest time checking the article thoroughly – after all, it will be carrying your name. Many experts find that, having looked through a drafted article, they prefer to rewrite most of it anyway.

Leaving ghost-writing to one side, the first time that you receive an edited version of something that you have written for an agency, you may think that there has been some sort of mistake. The article returned to you may only bear a passing resemblance to the one that you submitted! The role of editing in agency circles is very different from that for journals. As well as ensuring that your article reads well and is appropriate for the anticipated audience, the agency editor must make sure that the text fits the space allocated exactly, meets the marketing brief of his client and conforms to the house style of either the agency or the client company. House-style rules apply to wording, phraseology and the layout of articles. They may seem petty, but are necessary in publishing circles, as they enforce some sort of standardization on a company's products. You will probably never notice the effects of 'house styling', but if you find that something you have written has been changed consistently but for apparently no reason (e.g. if each time 'especially' appeared in your manuscript, it has been changed to 'particularly'), it is likely to be the result of editing into house style.

So, you have the edited version of your article in your hand. The best approach is to try to read the article as if it was a completely new piece of work. Does it make sense? Is it accurate? Does it flow well? Invariably, you will think that your original version was better, but if you can answer 'yes' to the preceding questions, there is probably little reason to make a fuss. However, on occasion you may find that the article no longer makes sense or you will spot inaccuracies that have been introduced. Most editors have science degrees, many have a PhD, but few, if any, have specialist medical knowledge. Their work is based on your original article, so if they have completely misinterpreted something then perhaps it was not clear in the first place!

A good editor will know when he is confused and will incorporate queries into the text for you to answer. Always answer these as clearly as possible, no matter how obvious the answer may appear to you. If you have real concerns about your article, talk to your editor and try to reach a compromise. If you are still unhappy, contact the account manager and suggest that another editor look at what has been done. If you still cannot reach a compromise,

check **proofs thoroughly** for **medical accuracy**

Table 6

Standard proof-correction marks

Text	Margin	
it is̶	ᶘ|	Delete letter/word that is crossed through
it/said	is⟋	Insert words at point marked in text
it is	∿/	Make text bold
it is	(ital)	Make text italic
(it is)	(Rom)	Make text Roman
it͟is	#⟋	Insert a space
10₂	⅄	Make marked text superscript
CO2̂	⋏	Make marked text subscript
⌊is⌋it⌋	(trs)	Transpose letters or words marked in text
it͟is	(stet)	Leave text as is

investigate the ease with which you can withdraw from the project (this will depend on any agreement you have made with either the agency or the pharmaceutical company).

Mark your comments clearly on to the manuscript using blue ink – your comments will be visible and the pages will also photocopy well. Print or use capitals if your handwriting is at all unclear. Using standard proof-correction marks in the margin will help the editor to interpret your amendments accurately (Table 6). Do not waste time tweaking or twiddling with sentences as it is likely that these changes will be ignored. The odd word is bound to be missing here and there – if you notice it, mark it up, but do not panic – your article will be subject to many more rounds of editorial checks. Most importantly, check that any Greek symbols are still correct (μg has a particular tendency to default to mg), decimal points are correctly placed and that any abbreviations or acronyms have been expanded accurately (particularly those relating to drug regimens). Also check the layout of all tables thoroughly. If you have been sent rough artwork to check, examine it for anatomical and labelling accuracy.

Your amended version may now be sent to the pharmaceutical company for comments; it is also likely that another editor will review it. As a result, you may be sent a further edited version and/or a further set of queries (this is why it is so important to find out who looks at what, and when, before committing yourself). When everyone is happy with the manuscript, a set of page proofs will be produced. This process is fraught with editorial dangers and you should check page proofs thoroughly (Table 7). If the errors on the proofs are a cause for concern, ask your editor to send you a revised set of pages to check. Often, the first page proofs will be the last opportunity you get to check your work. Mark any amendments very, very clearly and always keep a copy. Then sit back and wait to receive a copy of the glossy final product and, of course, your cheque!

Table 7

Checking page proofs

Check that:
- the text is complete and in the correct order
- Greek and/or mathematical symbols are correct
- drug regimens are correct
- figures are correctly placed (are slides/photographs correctly oriented?) and labels are accurately positioned

Unless you spot an inaccuracy:
- do not change the text or figures
- do not add extra text or figures

Mark your comments clearly, and indicate amendments with a cross in the margin. Make a copy of the pages for your files

---

Working with a publishing company

There are two routes into the world of publishing. You may be commissioned to write a book or chapter, or you may have an idea for a medical book that you would like to pursue. Again, if approached by a commissioning editor, you should find out exactly what is involved and what your royalty will be before committing yourself. Generally, writing a book will not generate a huge income. Most authors approach publishing as a means of disseminating their expertise to a wider audience and, of course, raising their profile and establishing a reputation; the royalty cheque is an added bonus.

Be aware that many medical publishers sell bulk quantities of their titles to pharmaceutical companies. Although this will obviously have a considerable effect on your royalty payment, realize that, in return, the pharmaceutical company may have their name printed on the front or back cover of the book. They will also be given the opportunity to review the manuscript and/or page proofs, and may comment accordingly. Check with your editor how much weight should be given to these comments – you will normally be free to take them on board or ignore them as you see fit. If this is not the case, you may not want to be involved with the project. For most publishers, producing a quality publication that will be valued by the reader is their priority.

If you agree to write the book, you will be sent a contract. Read it thoroughly – if any clauses cause concern, discuss them with your commissioning editor. Another good idea is to have a word with other authors who have worked with the publishing company in question – if you do not know of anyone yourself, ask the company for a few names.

If you have a startlingly good idea for a book, send an outline and details of the proposed audience to commissioning editors of medical publishing houses. And then wait! It has to be said, however, that few medical books start life in this way.

Publishing is a time-consuming business. Try to get an idea of the approximate schedule from the commissioning editor at the outset, but always be prepared for delays, particularly when several authors are involved. Keep the project moving and try to meet the deadlines.

Editing

If you are the editor or joint editor on a project, then your role may involve:

- suggesting authors for chapters
- approaching authors for contributions (or at least agreeing that letters be sent out in your name)

- suggesting a structure/chapter running order for the book or journal
- reviewing submitted chapters for suitability in terms of content and medical accuracy
- reviewing the whole publication for medical accuracy and clarity.

Although it may be tempting to do so, do not waste time laboriously correcting non-medical spelling mistakes and poor grammar. Your publisher's editor will do this. Concentrate on 'the big picture' and ask yourself whether the message is conveyed clearly and concisely to the audience you have in mind.

Further reading

Albert T. *Medical Journalism: The Writer's Guide*. Oxford: Radcliffe Medical Press, 1992.

Albert T. *Winning the Publications Game: How to get Published without Neglecting your Patients*. Oxford: Radcliffe Medical Press, 1996.

Benson J, Britten N. How much truth and to whom? Respecting the autonomy of cancer patients when talking to their families – ethical theory and the patients' view. *BMJ* 1996;313:729–31.

Buckman R. *How to Break Bad News: A Guide of Health Care Professionals*. Baltimore: Johns Hopkins University Press, 1992.

Buckman R, Kason Y. *How to Break Bad News – A Practical Guide for Healthcare Professionals*. London: Macmillan, 1993.

Evans H. *Newsman's English*. London: Heinemann, 1992.

Fallowfield I. Giving sad and bad news. *Lancet* 1993;341:476–8.

Faulkner A. *When the News is Bad. A Guide for Health Professionals*. Nelson Thornes, 1998.

Goodman NW, Edwards MB. *Medical Writing: A Prescription for Clarity*. Cambridge: Cambridge University Press, 1991.

Gunning R. *The Technique of Clear Writing* (revised edition). New York: McGraw Hill, 1971.

Kieffer GD. *The Strategy of Meetings*. London: Judy Piatkus, 1988.

Maquire P. Can communication skills be taught? *Br J Hospital Med* 1990;43:215–16.

Meredith C, Symonds P, Webster L *et al.* Information needs of cancer patients in the west of Scotland. *BMJ* 1996;313:724–6.

Northouse P, Northouse LLO. Communication and cancer: issues confronting patients, health professionals and family members. *J Psychosoc Oncol* 1987;5:17–45.

Novack DH, Plumer R, Smith RI *et al.* Changes in physician's attitudes toward telling the cancer patient. *JAMA* 1979;241:879–900.

O'Connor M. *Writing Successfully in Science.* London: HarperCollins, 1991.

O'Donnell M. Write for Money. In: *How to Do It.* Vol 2. London: BMJ, 1997.

Oken D. What to tell cancer patients. *JAMA* 1961;175:1120–8.

Silverman J, Kurtz S, Draper J. *Skills for Communicating with Patients.* Oxford: Radcliffe Medical Press, 1999.

Smith AJ, Preston D. Communications between professional groups in an NHS Trust hospital. *J Manage Med* 1996;10:31–9.

Effective communication

crisis management

"Smooth seas do not make skilled sailors"
African proverb

Although crises in medicine are much more common than in the airline business, airline personnel receive far more training in crisis management than doctors do. Learning to cope with and learn from crises is now an essential skill for a successful doctor. Litigation and other forms of conflict are becoming increasingly common in the NHS, and indeed throughout the world. One reason for this is undoubtedly poor-quality interpersonal working relationships. Part of the problem is that medical schools do not always teach students how to put medicine into practice and learn when mistakes are made.

Besides clinical ability, there are a number of key components of good clinical practice.

- You should practice sound clinical management. This is not only clinical ability, but means sticking to your own area of expertise and avoiding the temptation to cut corners.
- Competent administration is integral to good clinical practice. Be proactive; chase the results of investigations and defaulters to make sure that those with abnormal results are followed up.
- Clear communication is essential, including the keeping of accurate, up-to-date records.
- Apart from being clinically competent, a good doctor must be able to break bad news, provide counselling, obtain consent from patients for any form of intervention and generally deal kindly, professionally and effectively with people.

The difference between a consultant and a trainee is that the ultimate responsibility stops with the consultant in all of these regards. Good clinical practice and effective interpersonal skills will avert most potential crises.

Complaints from patients or relatives

When something goes wrong and patients complain, it is very often because one or more of the following three key points have not been dealt with effectively:

- counselling
- consent
- breaking bad news.

It is usually problems at these levels that escalate towards litigation. When someone complains, they usually want:

- an explanation
- an apology
- rectification.

An explanation and an apology do not necessarily mean admission of guilt. The most important point here is to put a human face on the problem and to see it from the other person's point of view. The reasons may be clear to you, and it may not have been anybody's fault, but nonetheless an unfortunate outcome deserves an explanation and an

an apology is not an admission of guilt

apology, if only on compassionate grounds. Often a problem can be mitigated by reassuring the patient that the same thing won't happen again to somebody else. It is only occasionally that patients demand financial recompense or blood. In short, do not assume that a patient complains because he is planning to sue you for everything you've got; often the complainant simply wants to know why something happened, to hear that you regret the outcome even if it was unavoidable at the time, and to be reassured that steps will be taken to ensure that it doesn't happen again. If necessary, advice from a medicolegal specialist should be sought (see pages 121–32).

Obviously, crisis management should be avoided if at all possible. Address issues before they have the opportunity to become crises, while there is more time for information to be gathered, to prepare an appropriate response and to communicate that response effectively. There are certain characteristics that typify medical crises:

- someone is to blame, either erroneously or maliciously, for the situation

- there is something important at stake
- a situation is brought into the open.

Clearly, certain aspects of medicine, such as working in an intensive care unit, have potential crises as part of everyday practice. However, crises that are possibly reproachable with legal action are likely to be those in which something has gone wrong. Whatever the cause, a crisis is an atypical occurrence that demands an immediate response, often in the face of insufficient information and evidence. Learn to recognize the traits and weaknesses that can lead to mistakes (Table 8). In such situations, interpersonal skills are tested acutely.

Unfortunately, litigation is now much more common than ever before. As the level of dissatisfaction rises among hospital employees, it is inevitable that patients will be influenced by the subsequent atmosphere. Media coverage of medical 'disasters' often compounds this problem. Patients have higher expectations than ever before, and are not afraid to complain if these are not met.

Table 8

Causes of medical mistakes

Organizational
- Weak leadership
- Education/research undervalued
- Cliques and factions present
- Lack of coherent strategy
- Poor communication
- Sparse infrastructure

Personal
- Defensive attitude in the face of criticism
- Inability to learn from mistakes
- Fortress mentality
- Poor collaboration
- Lack of skills
- Bad teamwork
- Poor motivation and attitude

Dealing with crises

The most important rule is to put a human face on the problem. The situation demands sympathy, understanding and, when a mistake has been made, an apology. Importantly, an expression of regret ('I'm terribly sorry this has happened') is not an admission of guilt. It is equally important to deal with the individual's perceptions ('I can see how this must seem to you') and not just the facts. Finally, as a doctor, you should remain polite, honest, caring and dignified at all times. Responding aggressively and defensively ('It's not my fault') is a very destructive way of dealing with such a situation. It is also vital for the whole team to learn from the mistake.

Risk management

The possibility that an adverse event has arisen because of a more fundamental problem should always be considered. This is the essence of 'risk management'. By monitoring and learning from all unusual, unintentional or adverse events and looking for patterns in their occurrence, potential crises may be averted. Only when effective risk management exists will you be able to reassure those around you that any crisis is a one in a million occurrence in an otherwise excellent track record. Remember the important dictum that 'people may come and go but a safety culture must prevail'.

Coping with violence

Most day-to-day violence encountered in medicine is verbal or threatened rather than physical. A dissatisfied patient may occasionally be verbally abusive, and it is important to have help to prevent the situation escalating. The presence of a third independent person, if only to corroborate your version of events at a subsequent enquiry, is important. If you are unsure how to respond to a verbally abusive patient, relative or member of staff, it is best to say nothing as any response might fuel their anger. Faced with silence, most people eventually run out of steam and begin to feel foolish. Never touch an abusive person as any form of body contact may be construed as assault, however well meaning your intention.

Nevertheless, your duty does not extend to having to tolerate abuse of any kind. If an attempt at reasonable discussion fails, then quietly, politely, but firmly terminate the interview as soon as possible, document the occurrence and inform the risk manager for the hospital Trust of the events, ideally with corroboration from an independent witness. If the person concerned is a patient, notify their GP of events and suggest that the patient be referred elsewhere.

Real physical violence in hospitals is comparatively rare, at least in western Europe. Threatened physical violence by angry patients or by patients who are under the influence of drugs or alcohol is much more common. Broadly speaking there are two situations: the first is when the patient is in need of urgent medical attention in which case care should be given despite the patient's behaviour, assuming of course that it is possible to administer treatment. In

> **document** all **threatening** and **abusive encounters**

the other scenario, the patient is physically threatening and not in urgent need of medical care or indeed of any treatment at all. Sometimes you may feel that enduring verbal abuse and physically threatening behaviour is part of your duty as a doctor, but you are under no obligation to do so and, if necessary, the patient can be physically removed from the hospital. However, you are obliged to point out any medical problem to the patient or to his family doctor to ensure that it is dealt with in due course.

If the patient is threatening but not under the influence of drugs or alcohol, generally, it is best to do nothing. If you remain seated and quiet, saying and doing nothing, sooner or later most patients will calm down. Never become physically threatening yourself – this only makes the situation worse. If the patient needs to be restrained, always involve hospital security staff or the police who are trained in the proper techniques – your job is to treat the patient. All hospitals now have 'risk managers' and security staff to deal with such situations.

Difficult colleagues

You can choose your friends, but you cannot choose your blood relatives or colleagues. Many so-called 'difficult colleagues' are simply people you would not choose to associate with socially. Nonetheless, they may have their own circle of professional friends who would view you similarly. On the other hand, many hospitals have a 'difficult' employee who seems to be a law unto himself. Such people usually continue to act in this way because no one has ever discussed with them the fact that their behaviour might be considered inappropriate – assuming that they are indeed a cause for concern beyond being mildly eccentric. Reasons for talking to a colleague about his conduct include:

- excess alcohol consumption
- drug abuse
- actions that affect the health and safety of others
- behaviour that may be offensive or embarrassing to others.

Some people are unaware of the effect their behaviour has on others. When an individual is confronted with this issue, he may respond with a torrent of abuse or aggression. Usually, the best course of action is to confront the individual, bring your concerns to his attention and then attempt to address the issues. Attempting to resolve such a situation with a sympathetic discussion is highly preferable to allowing it to escalate. It is a question of being assertive rather than aggressive. Although such a discussion potentially may be unpleasant, if conducted politely and in an even-handed manner, it is often productive.

If a colleague's behaviour continues to be a problem, particularly if substance abuse or anything that may be potentially harmful professionally is a factor, then you should inform the appropriate person, such as a clinical director or medical director of the Trust. Your comments about colleagues must be honest. It is better to act and stand by a colleague as a friend than to feel that the best way of supporting them is not to report the issue. The safety of patients must be your priority at all times. Your primary duty is to your patients and other colleagues for any such professional breach of conduct at work.

Sexual harrassment

One person may feel that certain behaviour constitutes sexual harassment while another individual may consider the same 'a piece of harmless fun'. In any relationship with patients or colleagues, you should attempt to see how your words and actions might be perceived. While most doctors are careful to consider this in their interactions with patients, they are often less observant in their relationships with colleagues. While many comments are intended as 'a bit of a laugh', they may not be interpreted as such by the recipient. If an individual fails to notice how badly their actions or words are received, further actions or words simply make matters worse.

Many victims of sexual harassment tolerate it. Indeed, they may even find it amusing in small doses, and laugh about it with their colleagues; however, it is never a good idea to tolerate such behaviour because sooner or later someone will be upset or offended. It is better to confront the individual concerned or alternatively report him to a third party who can take independent action. Such action might be simply to draw the matter to the attention of the wrongdoer who may then desist thereafter. Indeed, some people are horrified to find that they are

> it is **never** a
> **good idea** to **tolerate**
> **sexual harrassment**

perceived in this way when they genuinely felt they were being 'friendly and amusing'. More serious cases should be dealt with always by a clinical or medical director. Such people should be reminded that it is not what they mean by what they say or do but how others perceive it that is important.

If you are accused of sexual harassment, what should you do? Accusations often arise from one of two situations. A patient may accuse you of harassment because they feel that you behaved inappropriately during a history taking or physical examination. For example, vaginal examination or examination of the breasts may seem inappropriate to a patient who has come to see you with backache. If you can justify your behaviour, have kept careful notes and were simply being thorough then there is unlikely to be a problem. It is possible that the patient was seen by a senior house officer or registrar, but if your name, as consultant, was on the door you will need to discuss it with the individual in person. The alternative situation is that a patient may interpret your behaviour as inappropriate based on their own perception of events, in which case it is important to view the incident from the other person's perspective. If accused of sexual harassment, often the immediate reaction is to attempt to justify one's actions or otherwise talk your way out of the situation. The correct approach is to apologize profusely to the person your behaviour has offended and to undertake not to behave in such a way again.

If you are accused of more serious acts of sexual harassment that may contravene the standards of good behaviour set by the GMC, it is often best to say nothing until you have spoken with the medical or clinical director, your defence union or, in some cases, consulted your solicitor.

Racial and sexual discrimination

As everybody knows, racial and sexual discrimination are illegal. Although the law sets the standards by which we are expected to live, we are all aware that, in practice, these are regularly breached. Sometimes discrimination is used as a justification for someone not achieving a particular goal, when in fact they simply weren't up to the job. Irrespective of racial or gender issues, favouritism has always existed. In our dealings with others, we should try to be fair as we would not wish to be subject to such bias.

Nowadays, anybody who is involved in interview processes will be obliged to take a course in which matters of racial and sexual discrimination are addressed. Participants will be 'trained' not to discriminate against applicants on the grounds of race, sex, religion, or anything else for that matter. Application forms are being designed increasingly to exclude discrimination so far as is possible.

Dealing with the media following a crisis

After a recent spate of highly publicized medical disasters, it is certainly appropriate to consider how you would respond in such a circumstance. One unfortunate incident can spark a frenzy of antagonistic media interest, destroying staff commitment that has been built up over many years, literally overnight.

If such a situation arises, it is essential first to establish the facts surrounding the case and obtain group support. Everyone involved in the incident should meet to develop a common understanding of what exactly has taken place and how it should be handled. It is vital to create a united bond over any issue that attracts press attention, otherwise the press may attempt to generate fear of a witch-hunt, encouraging staff to get their individual defensive positions on record early. Elect a spokesperson, preferably someone who has had media training or experience, to deal with the press openly and honestly. Most Trusts have a designated press officer for precisely this reason. Elicit their support early on. Never attempt to go it alone.

Be wary about unsolicited telephone calls from journalists. Before answering their questions, try to find out what they know, where they got their information from and what their slant is. If possible, get your secretary to find out as much as possible about the journalist before agreeing to call him back out of clinic hours. If you do speak to journalists, always begin by giving some sound, positive information about how the organization works, thus providing evidence that the unit normally works well and effectively. Use other authoritative sources, such as Royal Colleges and specialist associations, to corroborate your position.

There is a tendency for doctors to bury their heads when it comes to media involvement. If you do not seize the opportunity to put good, positive news about clinical practice into the public domain, the public will only ever hear the bad news and all the good work that we do will be discounted.

Final thoughts

Crises are better avoided than managed once they have arisen. To avoid them, it is essential to develop a mindset in which you learn not only from your own but also from others' mistakes. The NHS will certainly have to change, focusing more proactively on learning from experience. Beliefs, attitudes and values that nurture a culture of blame and superficial analysis currently allow the same mistakes (such as wrongly administered spinal injections) to recur repeatedly. It is clear that, in the vast majority of cases, the cause of serious failure reaches far beyond the actions of the individuals directly involved. Attempts to develop a positive safety culture in medicine are now underway. Clinical governance is central to these efforts. This is the subject of the following chapter.

Further reading

Association of Trust Medical Directors. *When Things go Wrong – Practical Steps for Dealing with the Problem Doctor.* Hingsway Cheadle: British Association of Medical Managers, 1997.

Barach P, Small SD. Reporting and preventing medical mishaps: lessons from non-medical near-miss reporting systems. *BMJ* 2000;320:753–63.

Harpwood V. *Medical Negligence and Clinical Risk: Trends and Developments.* London: Monitor Press, 1998.

Kohn LT, Corrigan JM, Donaldson MS, eds. *To Err is Human: Building a Safer Health System.* Washington DC: National Academy Press, 1999.

Peason JT. Understanding adverse events: human factors. In Vincent CA, ed. *Clinical Risk Management.* London: BMJ Publications, 1995.

Simanowitz A. Accountability. In Vincent CA, Ennis M, Audley RJ, eds. *Medical Accidents.* Oxford: Oxford University Press, 1993:209–21.

The Department of Health. *Supporting doctors, protecting patients. A consultation paper on preventing, recognising and dealing with poor clinical performance of doctors in the NHS in England.* London: DOH, 1999.

clinical **governance** and **self-regulation**

"Every patient who is treated in the NHS wants to know that he can rely on receiving high quality care when needed. Every part of the NHS and everyone that works in it should take responsibility for working to improve quality."
The New NHS, Modern, Dependable,
Department of Health, 1997

Clinical governance is all about quality. Until recently, quality in hospital medicine was largely related to professional self-regulation; doctors did their best and quality was the result. Now, however, this has changed. Public expectation is considerably higher than ever before. The general level of dissatisfaction with the NHS is rising, and there have been highly publicized incidents in Bristol, Kent and at the Alder Hey that have shaken public faith in the profession further still. Consequently, the government is no longer happy to rely on professional self-regulation to ensure that quality standards are maintained. In fact, 'quality' itself has become an issue in recent years. In an attempt to improve the overall quality of the experience of patients undergoing medical care, the previous Conservative government introduced 'charter standards' without directly addressing the clinical issues. Various other initiatives to improve quality in clinical practice have been undertaken, such as the Confidential Enquiry into Perioperative Death, an initiative started by the Royal College of Surgeons some years ago. Indeed the whole issue of audit was introduced to improve outcomes, and clinical outcomes in particular.

Quality has always been a major issue. So what has changed? The present government introduced its plans for the health service in a document entitled *The New NHS: Modern, Dependable*. Quality issues were the central theme of the subsequent document, *A First Class Service: Quality in the New NHS*. In the original government timetable, clinical governance was to be established in 1999; the Trusts reported back in 2000, showing how this has been achieved. At the same time, the National Institute for Clinical Excellence (NICE) and the Commission for Health Improvement (CHI) were established and the idea of National Service Frameworks was promulgated.

The aim is to establish a national standard for quality for each and every major (and many minor – but expensive) clinical condition, hence the National Service Frameworks. NICE is responsible for ensuring that national standards are set, while CHI will monitor the standards regionally. Within each hospital Trust, it is the chief executive's responsibility to ensure that clinical governance is in place to achieve these standards which are set nationally and monitored regionally. In each Trust, a 'clinical governance group' will be responsible for ensuring that each directorate is doing what it should. The intention is for the entire process to be multidisciplinary, involving 'clinical teams'. Furthermore, patients' views should also be taken into account. The National Framework for Assessing Performance will evaluate clinical performance from the patient's perspective and the Annual National Survey of Patients and User Experience will determine whether clinical services meet the patients' needs. The work and bureaucracy involved in all of this is potentially staggering.

Defining clinical governance

What does clinical governance actually mean? *A First Class Service* defines clinical governance as 'a framework through which NHS organizations are accountable for continuously improving the quality of their services and safeguarding high standards of care by creating an environment in which excellence in clinical care will flourish'. This carries both clinical and organizational obligations. Indeed, the cynic might feel that the real motive behind clinical governance is to ensure that doctors meet organizational obligations to the Trust that employs them (and subsequently to the government), as well as their traditional professional and statutory obligations to their colleges and specialist associations.

The pillars of clinical governance

Some aspects of clinical governance are already familiar: audit is established and relevant; risk management is important, albeit less familiar to doctors (but familiar to nurses); and staff development is another well-established feature. These have been expanded into five 'pillars' of clinical governance:

- clinical audit
- clinical effectiveness
- clinical risk management
- quality assurance
- staff development.

The principal difference in the way that these aspects are being approached in clinical governance is that the 'team' is now the focus rather than the doctor; and the entire 'clinical experience' is being addressed rather than patients' treatment by the doctor specifically. So all points of contact between the hospital and the patient – sometimes referred to as 'the patient journey' – are addressed. It includes out-patients in the accident and emergency department, the ambulance service, the admission process, the ward as a physical environment, the domestic services, the nursing care, the care provided by other healthcare professionals and the medical care; every aspect is taken into account. The 'team' includes doctors, nurses, physiotherapists, dietitians, pharmacists, secretaries and anyone responsible for a particular 'clinical experience'.

Clinical audit

Doctors have been involved in clinical audit for sometime, although many specialties have never taken it very seriously. In clinical audit, performance within a given area is monitored and compared with others' performances; reasons that account for this difference are then identified. A mechanism can then be put in place to improve performance,

audit must address all the important quality issues

and reassessment should confirm that a better outcome has been achieved. Audit in hospitals has so far been entirely clinical. Doctors have worked out the best ways to approach and report the audit they wanted to undertake. In future, hospital managers will want to be assured that audit topics are comprehensive and the activities selected for audit in each directorate are systematic. Audit must address all the important quality issues, with the goal of improved overall quality of care, with particular reference to patient experience and outcome. In other words, it must be more open and accountable to outsiders.

Clinical effectiveness

Recent interest in effectiveness has centred on evidence-based clinical practice. A number of books and databases – particularly the Cochrane databases – have developed around the theme of evidence-based medicine. Clearly, the idea is very sound. There is no point in providing a treatment, particularly an invasive procedure, if it is ineffective, however well it is administered. Evaluating clinical effectiveness will ensure that ineffective treatments are identified and discontinued, and effective treatments are administered to the highest possible standard. One way of achieving this is to make sure that patients follow so-called 'care pathways', and that outcomes are monitored against the accepted national standards referred to previously.

Critics argue that much of the evidence obtained in this way is not 'medicine-based evidence'. Although evidence-based medicine is all very well for clear-cut medical problems in uncomplicated cases, this is often not the case in real life. Indeed, many patients are excluded from the clinical trials on which evidence-based medicine is based for precisely this reason. 'Case mix' is therefore an important factor in the interpretation of clinical effectiveness, particularly when an external authority may judge a consultant on the outcome of his activities. It is argued that doctors will not want to treat complicated patients if they are to be judged by the same standards as those doctors who treat the straightforward cases. Clinical effectiveness in practice is not a case of simply monitoring morbidity and mortality, but by finding out whether treatments were appropriate and effective for a patient's specific clinical circumstances. There are many examples of treatment, in both medicine and surgery, that may occasion neither morbidity nor mortality, but which make no difference to the course or outcome of a clinical condition – usually at some considerable financial expense.

Clinical risk management

By recognizing and reviewing the adverse events that occur, ways to prevent them can then be identified. The goal of risk management is to reduce the occurrence and consequences of adverse events. For some time, risk management in hospitals has been associated with health and safety. Anything that is not a part of routine patient care or organizational activity is documented as an 'incident', and these incidents are analysed on a regular basis. The analysis serves to identify any underlying patterns that may suggest a more fundamental problem that needs to be addressed. A national reporting system has been proposed. Most incidents are relatively trivial, until an incident presents in a slightly different form so as to be termed a crisis. Incidents (within the definition given) can be identified by anybody working within an organization. On the whole, they tend to be reported by nurses who are in closer contact with patients and are much more familiar with the concepts of risk management and health and safety. Other points for consideration in risk management include specific points raised by patients, usually in letters

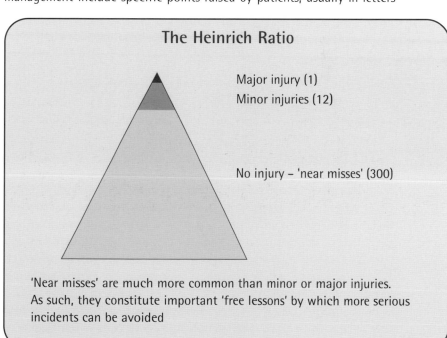

The Heinrich Ratio

Major injury (1)
Minor injuries (12)

No injury – 'near misses' (300)

'Near misses' are much more common than minor or major injuries. As such, they constitute important 'free lessons' by which more serious incidents can be avoided

of complaint. These need to be read, not just for the particular complaint, but as a means of identifying underlying problems that may be of a more serious nature.

The aim of clinical risk management is to apply these ideas more specifically to patient care. All members of the clinical team must be encouraged to identify and report adverse events – so-called 'free lessons' (see the Heinrich Ratio, page 93) – enabling everyone to learn from such experiences in a blame-free way. The ultimate goal is a reduced risk of adverse events, and therefore improved patient care. The most obvious clinical improvement would be a reduction in the incidence of iatrogenic disease, which has been estimated to cost the NHS more than £2 billion each year (Table 9).

Table 9

Estimated annual cost of iatrogenic disease to the NHS

- £2 billion due to lost bed days
- £400 million resulting from medical negligence claims
- 6600 device-related incidents reported
- 9800 serious drug reactions reported

Quality assurance

There is a considerable overlap between quality assurance and clinical effectiveness, and of course both are intimately involved in clinical audit. Quality assurance is principally concerned with the monitoring and measurement of performance against standards, rather than the less rigorous assessments of clinical audit. Quality assurance programmes are particularly important in screening programmes, pathology, blood transfusion and radiology. In clinical practice, good examples of quality assurance include proper practice in keeping patient records, prescribing and administering treatments appropriately, and completing diagnostic coding.

Clinical governance and self-regulation

Staff development

In many professions, staff development or continuing professional development, including a regular appraisal process, is standard and well established. Regular appraisals are now widely regarded as an integral part of getting the best out of the personnel of any business.

Until recently, staff development in the health service has largely been a passive process. A doctor was appointed to a post and stayed in it until the end of that particular appointment, when he moved on. Unless he was particularly good or particularly bad, nobody took much notice of his performance during that time. However, appraisals and assessments for trainees have been introduced, and consultants must provide evidence of continuing medical education to demonstrate that they are keeping abreast of recent developments. Poor performance has been brought to the forefront in cases such as that involving paediatric cardiac surgery in Bristol, illustrating that an adequate knowledge base on its own, which is probably the best that continuing medical education alone can provide, is insufficient. The consultant must have adequate clinical and non-clinical skills on

> **good performance** depends on **sufficient clinical** and **non-clinical skills**

which to draw if he is to provide a sufficiently good overall performance. In the case of a surgeon or interventionist, this includes both his technical operative skills and his intraoperative decision-making. Although all doctors have their own particular clinical skills, they also have non-clinical skills that are common to all specialties. In particular, these concern counselling, breaking bad news, communicating with patients and staff, dealing with problems and relating well with other people. These interpersonal skills are probably more important to an average patient than the clinical skills. Likewise, poor clinical performance is not just performing an operation badly or giving the wrong drug dose or treatment, but also poor record-keeping, poor communication, disruptive working behaviour or simply the inability to work as part of a team.

The 'job plan' is a tool used to identify what a consultant actually does. Completed annually, it has simply documented the average working

The Bristol cardiac surgery case

The Bristol case involved a team of cardiac surgeons working in Bristol and concerned their performance of a particular type of 'switch' surgery used for the treatment of a specific congenital malformation. This operation was established as the standard of care, but in order to achieve consistently good results, a very high standard of surgical technique is required together with scrupulous pre-operative evaluation and postoperative care. A national register of these operations had been established sometime before and so the overall mortality was known as a baseline against which individual results could be judged.

It had become apparent that the results in Bristol were substantially worse (mortality was double that of other units) than the national register suggested they should be and it also became apparent that the parents of the children involved had been given unrealistic expectations of what surgery could achieve. Furthermore, although the results at Bristol had been pointed out to various 'authorities' and to the surgeons themselves, the surgeons had continued to operate and no effective action had been taken to deal with the issues that had arisen.

This raised a number of issues in relation to clinical standards and audit by which an individual surgeon's results can be compared against a generally accepted national standard: how an individual doctor's personal performance is monitored and by whom; the responsibility of an individual consultant in relation to his own performance; the honesty with which risks are explained to patients; and the need to protect patients from doctors who are 'in difficulty' (in any sense of the word) let alone how to assess technical expertise and clinical competence, particularly in advanced procedures. The latter has obvious knock-on effects with respect to training; how can doctors work competently while on the inevitable 'learning curve' which accompanies undertaking new procedures, and how should doctors be trained to perform difficult advanced procedures which are not part of routine practice? The Royal Colleges, specialist associations and individual NHS Trusts are currently trying to address these issues.

Clinical governance and self-regulation

week of a consultant – ward rounds, out-patient clinics, operating lists and other 'fixed sessions' plus on-call duties, administration, research, audit, examining, teaching and committee attendance. In the past, this has been completed by the consultant and signed off by his clinical director. In future, however, this is likely to change. 'Continuing professional development' will probably involve annual appraisal of each consultant by his clinical director or other nominated individual; the job plan, continuing medical education and other governance-related activities (audit and clinical effectiveness) will probably form a focus of this interview. This may be viewed as a procedure aimed primarily at identifying and reporting poor performance. Although this is undoubtedly one reason for this exercise, there is nonetheless a positive side to clinical professional development. It must be remembered that identifying poor performance is a valuable goal in itself, particularly if it prevents harm.

Revalidation of doctors' registration

In 1998, the GMC decided that doctors must demonstrate, on a regular basis, that they are up to date and fit to practice in their chosen field. Doctors who fail to show this competence will lose their registration.

The revalidation of registration is the biggest single change to medical regulation since the Medical Act, set by the GMC in 1958. As a result, the medical register has become a record of a doctor's continuing fitness to practice rather than a historical record of qualifications acquired in training. Although doctors' revalidation will be recorded centrally and publicly through the GMC's registers, quality assurance of an individual's performance will be monitored at a local level.

The precise details of how to deliver revalidation are subject to detailed discussion at the time of publication. There are many sensitive issues, in particular whether it is right for NHS management to become deeply involved in assessing the clinical skills and knowledge of doctors. The combination of revalidation and managerial quality assurance, such as clinical governance, promises to reassure the public that robust systems are in place to monitor and support doctors in their work. These systems also serve to demonstrate that the majority of doctors, who are both able and conscientious, reach the high standards required of them.

Playing your part

At this stage, the most important thing to do is get involved with the clinical governance programme being developed by your Trust and your directorate. Work together with all your colleagues, looking at what you do together, how you do it and how well you do it.

Deaths and complications meetings are a good channel for focusing on clinical problems, but remember to focus on all aspects of these problems. Take particular note of nursing and other paramedical activities, adverse incidents and patient complaints. Find out what you can do to reduce the risk of all adverse events.

Evidence-based best practice should be identified. Audit your activities to make sure best practice is followed and national standards of performance achieved. Aim to identify and discontinue ineffective treatments or other wasteful practices. When problems of an organizational or managerial nature arise, make hospital management aware. This includes faulty equipment, insufficient staffing, poor hospital fabric and any other organizational aspect that adversely affects clinical practice.

Within the framework of clinical governance itself, the single biggest barrier is adequate information. This is closely followed by increasingly insufficient time to process and analyse this information. It is certainly true that for sophisticated analysis and results that will stand up to rigorous external scrutiny, information technology in most Trusts is currently woefully inadequate. Nonetheless, most of the general points outlined here can be addressed without recourse to sophisticated information technology, and you are likely to benefit if the principles of clinical governance are approached with an open mind.

> get **involved** with the **clinical governance programme** at **your Trust**

Most importantly, remember that you are not working in splendid isolation but as part of a team, and that people around you will begin to take more of an interest in what you do than they ever have done before. Clinical governance is a train coming down the track. You could try to stop it by standing in the way, or you can move aside, but be left behind. The best policy is to leap aboard and make it one of the vehicles of your own as well as your individual institution's success.

Further reading

Burke C, Lugon M. Integrating clinical risk and clinical audit – moving towards clinical governance. *Healthcare Risk Resource* 1998;2:16–18.

Department of Health. *The New NHS. Modern, Dependable.* Cm 3807. London: DOH, 1997.

Department of Health. *A First Class Service: Quality in the New NHS.* London: DOH, 1998.

General Medical Council. *Revalidating Doctors: Ensuring Standards, Securing the Future.* London: GMC, 2000.

Lugon M, Secker-Walker J. *Clinical Governance: Making it Happen.* London: Royal Society of Medicine Press, 1999.

Miles A, Hampton J, Hurwitz B, eds. *NICE, CHI and the NHS Reforms: Enabling excellence or imposing control?* London: Key Advances, 2000.

management issues

Keith Parsons FRCS
Consultant Urological Surgeon, Past Chief Executive of the
Royal Liverpool University Hospitals NHS Trust

*"The physician must be prepared not only to do his
duty himself, but also to secure the cooperation
of the patient, of the attendants and of externals"*
Hippocrates' first aphorism

It is improbable that Hippocrates could have anticipated the management issues that doctors in the NHS are facing today, but undoubtedly he had sound advice for us when he spoke of the cooperation of 'externals'. As doctors, we are quick to see managers as externals. While the shrewd might nurture their cooperation, the most successful will collaborate willingly and readily in the management processes and structures that are crucial and pivotal components of a thriving hospital, primary care group or partnership practice. Always bear in mind that the principal concern of everyone involved in the delivery of health services must be the effective care, treatment and safety of patients.

The business of health

Whether we like it or not, the NHS of the year 2000 and beyond has to be a managed system. It is not a democracy and must actively avoid responding to only the strongest vested interest. In the past, the NHS has often been vulnerable to this. It has to meet the demands of elected government, which is in turn accountable to the electorate, and the needs of those who use the service. Currently, expenditure in the NHS accounts for 6.7% of the UK's gross domestic product and, although we may consider this amount to be inadequate for the demands placed upon it, this is still a colossal sum. Spending such amounts cannot be a random process, and knowing what is delivered and how, and the ways in which this can be improved, is the very essence of management. We should all contribute enthusiastically and energetically to this process if we are to retain the trust and cooperation of our patients.

How to manage

First, forget the word 'administration'; the NHS is too complex and important to be merely administered. Administration is a completely inadequate concept for modern healthcare. It breeds bureaucracy, slowness and pedantry, and stifles imaginative and innovative thinking. A hospital is a complex organization, of which a great number of people, including those treated by it and those who work for it, have a diverse range of requirements. Nowadays, most city hospitals employ the equivalent of the population of a small town and may see a total number of patients equivalent to the population of a provincial city each year. Indeed, if visitors are also taken into consideration, the number of people coming through the hospital doors each year may equal the population of Denmark! Consequently, an enormous range of diverse requirements are generated, from simple procurement functions to complex interactions of, for example, employment law, health and safety legislation, fire regulations, design technology, informatics and data protection, to name but a few. Each of these elements has no direct reference to medical interactions, yet all are vital in ensuring that patients receive the highest quality treatment. It is essential that all of these aspects are managed with authority and skill.

Not everybody is interested in management, but in the end it boils down to the fact that you either become involved or are managed by somebody else. Generally, it is better to be involved in it yourself.

Probably the most important management decisions concern:
- setting priorities
- planning to achieve them
- maintaining the quality of the service provided as a consequence.

It is impossible to underestimate the importance of quality. Put yourself in the place of a worried relative or sick patient, and you will quickly realize that a quality service is paramount, queues and delays are unacceptable, and an almost guaranteed outcome desirable. Viewing the NHS from a concerned relative's perspective will help you appreciate the importance of these factors.

Managing change

As the consultant lead of a clinical team, the clinical director in management, or indeed in any other area such as a professional association, remember the importance of informing people what is intended to bring about change, what purpose is served and remind them of their responsibilities during the changes. Similarly, when the changes have been brought about, remind others of what has been done and why. By keeping people well informed, they are more likely to

> get **involved** in **management** or **you** will have to be **managed**

comply because they feel involved. Your colleagues will generally be grateful that somebody else is doing the managing; however, be careful not to make them feel their opinions are not wanted. Keep talking to them throughout, reminding them collectively what is being done. A successful doctor/manager is a team builder, a motivator and an innovator.

Understanding the structure

A successful doctor should be familiar with the management structure of the NHS Trust in which he works. This will equip him with the necessary tools to effect change and improvements in patient care when needed, and enable him to foster a spirit of collaboration and cooperation. To get to grips with the management structure, it is important to understand the basic differences between executive and governance functions.

Management structures

Every NHS Trust is managed by a board of executive and non-executive directors, with every director of equal status. Executive directors are responsible for the day-to-day management of the Trust. Non-executive directors are key members of the local community appointed to the Trust board by the Secretary of State for Health. They must ensure that the executives perform their duties within the requirements of a public body, and in doing so, fulfil their governance function. The entire board sets the strategy for the Trust, and the Chief Executive must see that the strategy is

management structures vary from trust to trust

enacted, while the Trust chairman, a non-executive director, ensures that this process takes place. The chair is responsible directly to the Secretary of State, although regular contact with the NHS Executive is maintained through the regional chairman.

Below board level, each Trust has a slightly different management structure, within which each service discipline has a line-management responsibility to the Chief Executive and the Board. This management responsibility is different from the professional responsibility of doctors, which is determined by the GMC.

Most service disciplines are structured as clinical directorates with a Clinical Director who is responsible to the Chief Executive. Remember that clinical directors do an awful lot, but what they do not do is direct clinically! Many will have had some management training, but if an opportunity to become a clinical director arises, do not hold back from accepting if you have not had this preparatory experience.

Effective management

As a general rule, doctors should make good managers. Our very training requires us to respond immediately to potential clinical catastrophes with authoritative management. The discipline, clarity of thought and authority of action needed to approach the day-to-day situations in which doctors find themselves are not altogether different from the requirements of an effective manager.

A clinical manager must recognize that what is required is relatively simple. Workload, personnel and budget, the essence of all business plans whether for the biggest corporation or the smallest clinical directorate, have to be reconciled. The '*kiss*' principle certainly applies – Keep It Simple, Stupid!

Accountability

The Chief Executive is accountable, ultimately to Parliament, for the organization. This accountability is through the Chief Executive of the NHS, who is himself accountable through the system of Parliamentary Select Committees – either through the Parliamentary Select Committee on Health or the Public Accounts Committee. Until recently, a Trust Chief Executive's accountability extended only to three statutory financial duties:

- to achieve financial balance
- to meet a predetermined return on the capital asset of the Trust
- to operate within the external funding limit for the Trust.

The modern and dependable NHS has added another statutory function for which the Chief Executive is accountable – a responsibility for clinical governance. This does not involve any direct executive role in patient management, but is a requirement that ensures that all clinicians, not just doctors, deliver healthcare to the Trust's patients at a level required by a public body. Clinical governance is in its early days, and we all are still learning what that 'required level' might be. However, clinical governance certainly presents an opportunity for the

> **clinical governance** represents an **opportunity** for **healthcare professionals**

healthcare professions, which can be used in the context of continuous quality improvement, and the most successful will grasp its concepts eagerly (see *Clinical governance and self-regulation*, page 89).

Working with your manager colleagues

It is a grave mistake to underestimate the commitment of NHS managers to the healthcare service and the institutions in which they work. They are as important to successful patient care as any other professional group in the hospital. Generally, NHS managers have many years of experience and have worked extensively at different management levels in health authorities, hospitals and elsewhere. It is essential to remember that everyone is working towards a common goal.

The dangers of intellectual arrogance

To be considered inferior and then to demonstrate otherwise is a powerful and disarming weapon, one some managers will use readily. Always avoid assuming intellectual superiority – it is better never to run the risk of being caught in this simple trap and being made to look foolish.

Don't hide behind clinical imperative

It can be tempting to raise the clinical imperative argument to get your own way. 'My patients must have this or they will suffer appallingly' is a cry that has been heard all too commonly, but is often unjustified by the clinical circumstance. No doubt there are circumstances when you will make demands on behalf of your patient, but do so in an intelligent and thoughtful way that engages proper discussion. If you try the old technique of 'shroud waving', you will find that you only get away with it once or twice.

Money matters

You might be forgiven for thinking that money does not matter, but since the NHS became cash-limited, it does. We should therefore be as cost-efficient as possible in all that we do. Everything done for patients has a cost implication and we must ensure that maximum benefit is achieved for as many as possible. As politicians make the ultimate decision on total healthcare expenditure, they are responsible for rationing. It is the clinicians' responsibility to direct that expenditure; the more effectively and efficiently this is done, the better the management relationship will become.

Beware the zero-game argument

It is easy to assume that any development in a limited resource system has to be paid for by shifting resources from elsewhere and this is true, to some extent. But Paul doesn't always have to be paid by a robbed Peter. If you are innovative in your thinking, there are often ways to fund new developments that do not require simple transfer of money from one project to another. Be imaginative and discuss the alternatives with your manager colleagues; it is likely that you will find a most receptive ear. In industry, there are no doubt thousands of examples of very simple measures that have released resources. One of the most impressive was that of a worker at the Bryant and May matchbox company who suggested putting sandpaper on one side of the box only rather than both. This simple suggestion saved the company millions of pounds. There is no reason why similar suggestions should not apply in medicine. Those most likely to identify such initiatives are those working closest to patients.

Demand evidence-based management

Management is a sophisticated science and those working in this field are professionals. They will respect a legitimate challenge and you should demand the same standards from your management colleagues as you do from other medical professionals. It is not unreasonable to ask for evidence to support the management's propositions. Evidence will doubtless be provided, but the subsequent discussion will serve to focus both parties and ultimately enhance the outcome. A track record of working in this way will result in managers turning to you first when they need help making difficult decisions.

Take an interest in the contracting process

It is all too easy for doctors to stand back and let others struggle with the complexities of contracting, and then criticize the outcome. The advent of primary care groups is already making the contracting process between primary and secondary care more complicated than ever before. Words may change and sentiments alter, but there will always be a need for hospitals to determine what they can deliver and the demands from primary care to deliver more at a lower cost. Successful doctors will be interested in this process and assist wherever possible. Contracts and finance departments need help, so assist when you can. In this way, much of the nonsense seen in the past will be abolished.

There is a pressing need to understand the new relationship between hospitals and general practitioners, who will have more influence on policy and direction in the future. When the rationing debate is considered, this relationship will become ever more relevant.

Recognize corporate responsibility

There is only one NHS, for which we all work.

Conflicts of interest

In some cases, it will be impossible to meet both the needs of an individual patient and the patient population as a whole, and you may need to make decisions about use of resources and provision of patient care. Such dilemmas have no simple solution. When faced with these situations, you must consider the priorities of the government, the NHS and your Trust. As a clinician, however, the care of your patient must be your first concern, bearing in mind the consequences your decision will have on the available resources and the choices of other patients. Your responsibility as a manager and doctor is to allocate resources in a way that best serves the interests of the community or entire patient population. In both capacities, you will make the best decision by using the best evidence from research and audit.

Protecting patients from harm

As a doctor and manager, you must take action if you believe that patients are at risk of serious harm. Concerns about safety may arise from the results of critical incident reporting, clinical audit, complaints from patients or information provided by colleagues. If you receive such information, you have a duty to act on it. As a manager, it will be necessary for you to establish the facts before taking action yourself.

always take action if patients are at risk

Alternatively, you may need to report the concerns to your own manager or a senior colleague.

Dealing with colleagues

If your responsibilities include managing colleagues, ensure that procedures are in place for dealing with their concerns and that all staff are made aware of them. As a manager, you must be prepared to discuss problems that your staff encounter in their professional capacity both sympathetically and constructively. You must also be willing to take any necessary action should serious problems emerge. All concerns should be investigated, documented and, if genuine, acted upon following discussions with other colleagues and senior managers. The protection of patients should remain the driving force at all times.

Final thoughts

Politics are a fact of life in the NHS. Difficult as it may be to accept, both doctors and managers will always be subject to the frustrations of working in a politically driven and resource-limited healthcare delivery system. The best mechanism for dealing with this is to work together, recognizing and striving to meet the particular demands that the system creates. The alternative is to take entrenched opposing positions – this only wastes time and energy.

Perhaps the greatest satisfaction that a successful doctor can have is recognition of his worth, so take pride in your hospital and make the Board proud of you. Taking a pride in the institution in which you work is a good starting point. Behind the façade of league tables and benchmarking lies the real issue of working for and with your local team. This has wider implications from a strategic standpoint. If you get this right, everyone associated with your institution will take pride in the success that you achieve.

Further reading

Association of Trust Medical Directors. *When Things go Wrong – Practical Steps for Dealing with the Problem Doctor.* Hingsway Cheadle: British Association of Medical Managers, 1997.

Burrows M, Dyson R, Jackson P, Saxton H, eds. *Management for Hospital Doctors.* Oxford: Butterworth Heinemann, 1994.

Chantler C. How to be a manager. *BMJ* 1989;298:1505–8.

Chantler C. Management and information. *BMJ* 1992;304:623–5.

Drucker PF. *The Practice of Management.* London: Pan Books, 1968.

Drucker PF. *Managing the Non-Profit Organization.* New York: HarperCollins, 1990.

General Medical Council. *Maintaining Good Clinical Practice.* London: GMC, 1998.

Hadley R, Forster D, eds. *Doctor Managers – Experiences in the Front Line of the NHS.* London: Longman, 1993.

Harrison A, Dixon J. *The NHS: Facing the Future.* London: King's Fund Publishing, 2000.

Harrison EF. *The Managerial Decision Making Process.* Boston: Houghton-Mifflin, 1987.

Harrison S. NHS management. *NAHAT NHS Handbook 1996/97.* Section 1.5, 1997.

Harrison S. *Managing the National Health Service – Shifting the Frontier?* London: Chapman and Hall, 1998.

Heirs B, Farrell P. *The Professional Decision Thinker. Our New Management Priority.* London: Grafton, 1991.

Institute of Health Services Management. *How to Handle Complaints.* London: IHSM, 1998.

Light DW. The real ethics of rationing. *BMJ* 1997;315:112–15.

Lindenfield G. *Managing Anger.* London: Thorsons, 1993.

Millar B. Clinicians as managers: medics make their minds up. *Health Service J* 1991;21 February:17.

Nelson MJ. *Managing Health Professionals.* London: Chapman and Hall, 1989.

Spurgeon P, Barwell F. *Implementing Change in the NHS: A Practical Guide for Managers.* London: Chapman and Hall, 1991.

Turill T, Wilson D, Young K. *The Characteristics of Excellent Doctors in Management.* Thirl: NHS Management Executive, 1991.

UKCC. *Reporting Unfitness to Practice – Information for Employers and Managers.* London: UKCC, 1996.

Welbourne IWB. The management of change. *Br J Hosp Med* 1990;44:53–5.

White A. Managing the chair. In: *Management for Clinicians.* London: Edward Arnold, 1993.

White A. *Managing Meetings.* London: Churchill Livingstone, 1996.

White A, ed. *Textbook of Management for Doctors.* London: Churchill Livingstone, 1996.

Management issues

finance

Andrew CD Lang FCA
Sandison Lang & Co Chartered Accountants

"Annual income twenty pounds, annual expenditure nineteen pounds, nineteen shillings and six, result happiness. Annual income twenty pounds, annual expenditure twenty pounds ought and six, result misery."
Mr Micawber in *David Copperfield*

Traditionally, doctors have not really focused on financial matters very much. The assumption has always been that medicine is an intellectually and financially satisfying vocation. Many regard simply qualifying as a doctor as a guarantee of financial success; beyond that, they feel there is no need to worry about the slightly unsavoury issue of money.

In fact, the reverse is true: financial security breeds success and success breeds financial security. To begin on a good footing, always be scrupulously honest in financial and commercial matters related to your work. It is also important to avoid accumulating large debts.

There are, however, two exceptions for which it is acceptable to take on a debt, and they are taking on a student loan for training, and borrowing for a short overseas placement in the form of an elective while you are a student or junior doctor. A student loan enables you to qualify (final-year medical students in 1999 had an average debt of £7326); once this is achieved overseas visits can broaden your outlook, provide invaluable clinical experience and enhance your CV, giving selection committees something to discuss in your first crucial interviews. Beg, borrow, but do not steal the money needed for either or both of these!

The early years (post-qualification to consultant)

Following qualification, your first hospital appointment will provide a regular monthly salary; spending and saving wisely at this time will provide solid foundations for the future.

Buying property

Over the years, property has been regarded as one of the safest investments. Therefore, to maximize capital appreciation, the sooner you can step on to the property ladder, the better. Consider taking the largest possible mortgage at the outset; as your income rises, the mortgage repayments will represent a lower percentage of your net income. The three main options for repaying the mortgage are outlined in Table 10.

Renting property

Rental payments are often money wasted – the money could be put towards a mortgage. If your employment requires that you change location every year or so, as is often the case with junior doctors, you could rent out your property on a short-term basis to recoup the mortgage repayments. Hospital Trusts will often pay your removal expenses.

Long-term sickness/critical illness insurance

Under the terms of the NHS Superannuation Scheme, in the event of sickness or illness, you will receive:
- full salary for the first 6 months of incapacity
- half salary for the next 6 months.

After 1 year of permanent disability, the benefits depend on the number of years of NHS service, which are unlikely to be significant at this stage of your career. You would therefore be strongly advised to consider taking out your own sickness policy; the sooner you do this, the cheaper it will be. Sickness insurance with the benefits deferred for 6 months should, for a 30-year-old, cost no more than £15 per month for £10 000 per annum until the age of 60.

Table 10

Mortgages

Repayment mortgage
- The capital and interest are paid off over a period of years

Endowment mortgage
- A loan is taken out from a mortgage company and interest only is payable throughout the lifetime of the loan
- The loan is paid off from the proceeds of an endowment policy at the end of the fixed period
- An endowment policy running parallel with a mortgage is a long-term regular savings plan that also offers life insurance
- Each month the endowment policy holder invests money into the insurance company's long-term investment fund which, in turn, invests in a mixture of shares, government stock, company loans, property and other schemes
- At the start of the policy, there is an agreement to pay the premiums for a set period (usually 25 years)
- At the end of the set period or if premature death occurs, the insurance company hands over a guaranteed lump sum called the 'sum assured'

Single account which meets all banking and borrowing needs
- Your property is used as security for a borrowing facility that meets all personal financial needs. No more separate accounts for mortgages, credit cards, current accounts or loans – one account covers all
- You agree a borrowing facility based on the value of your house and your annual income
- Your salary and any other income is paid into the single account
- You must stay within the agreed borrowing facility and repay the borrowings by the time you retire
- You must have life insurance to cover the borrowing facility at all times

Taxation

There is no point in paying more tax than you need to. Always submit details of tax-deductible expenses (e.g. professional and medical defence subscriptions) to the Inland Revenue; if there is a requirement to provide certain medical items, such as medical equipment, under the terms and conditions of employment in the NHS, ensure a tax claim is submitted.

Wills

Make a will, having taken some professional advice. Many individuals die intestate, leaving their relatives the potentially divisive task of guessing their intentions. You cannot assume that the law will follow your own logic when it comes to distributing your legacy.

Financial advisors

Most financial advisors are paid on a commission basis – the more they sell, the more commission they earn. Fully accredited independent financial advisors will offer their services on an hourly fee basis, with commissions being returned should any insurance policy have been effected. Always try to find an advisor who works independently. There are advisors who specialize in working with doctors – find out if your colleagues have any recommendations.

The middle years (consultant)

With a consultant appointment comes your opportunity to move into private practice (see page 45). Find yourself an accountant who specializes in advising doctors. He will advise you on the minutiae of keeping accurate records and taxation issues.

Keeping records

It is essential that you regard your private practice as a business, and appreciate the need for accurate accounting records (Table 11) and regular reviews of income and expenditure.

Table 11

Finance in private practice

Organize

- A private practice bank account
- A separate credit card to cover incidental private practice expenditure (e.g. car and conference expenditure)

Keep

- A private practice petty-cash book that details practice cash expenditure (e.g. on stamps and small items of stationery)
- Full records of patient fees rendered
- The private practice patient appointments diary
- Accurate records of income and expenditure – complete the cheque book stubs and keep all invoices for expenditure*

*The law requires that all accounting records are maintained for a period of 6 years

Private practice accounts have to be submitted to the Inland Revenue for taxation purposes annually; taxation is paid on the ultimate net profits. In addition to the normal running costs of the practice, tax relief is available on capital items of expenditure, such as cars, equipment, fixtures, fittings and furnishings. A sample profit and loss sheet is shown in Table 12.

Beware of the tax implications when undertaking private practice from your home. Be sure to take sound financial advice regarding this point. If your house is classified as a business rather than simply a residence, in theory, you may be liable for capital gains on its appreciation.

Personal pensions

Consider investing in a personal pension. Most consultants who have enjoyed a financially rewarding private practice will be unable to maintain

Table 12

Sample private practice profit and loss account

		£	£
Income	Patient fees invoiced		95000
	Other fees (e.g. medicolegal)		4500
			99500
Expenses	Consulting room costs	6500	
	Secretary	7500	
	Drugs and medical purchases	500	
	Assistants' fees	1500	
	Medical Defence Union/Medical Protection Society	4500	
	Printing, postage, stationery	750	
	Office costs (e.g. computer-related)	250	
	Books and journals	250	
	Bank charges and interest	650	
	Telephone in consulting rooms	300	
	Accountancy fees	1000	
	Bad debts	1500	
	Telephone and mobile phones (the proportion used on practice business)	500	
	Car expenses (practice proportion)	2500	
	Use of house for professional purposes	750	
	Spouse's assistance	3000	
	Spouse's pension contributions	1500	
	Conferences/courses (less refunds)	700	
	Depreciation	4200	
			38350
Net profit for the year			61150

their standard of living on the NHS pension of approximately one-half of their final NHS salary. Invest the maximum amount annually (Table 13). From a tax point of view, there is no other type of investment for which you can get tax relief when you pay the money in, enjoy the benefits of a fund that pays no tax on its income and gains, and can take part of the fund as a lump sum that is not taxable.

invest in a
personal pension

The dos and don'ts of taxation

Complete the annual tax return form accurately and on time – failure to do this will automatically result in interest and penalties.

Have a financial 'health check' from time to time – discuss your affairs with an accountant or tax advisor. Don't get caught without money in the bank when your tax bill arrives. Save for annual tax liabilities on a monthly basis; as a rough guide, set aside approximately one-third of your gross professional income.

Table 13

Maximum contributions to a private pension based on 'net relevant earnings', with earnings cap at £91 800

Age at 6 April 2000 (years)	Proportion of income that can be invested into a private pension in the financial year 2000–2001
≤ 35	17.5
36–45	20
46–50	25
51–55	30
56–60	35
61–74	40

Remember that tax legislation is subject to a review in the Chancellor's budget, and the law may change. Before you carry out any tax planning that will affect your situation in future years, ask yourself:

- how much the various forms of tax relief are worth to you
- how you could rearrange your affairs if the law was changed and the current forms of relief were curtailed or abolished.

Treat tax advice given over a gin and tonic sceptically. Very often, a friend or colleague does not understand all the ramifications of his own tax affairs, let alone yours.

Be scrupulously honest and transparent about your financial affairs. Before you take any action, ask yourself whether you would be happy for all your tax affairs to be scrutinized by a tax inspector. Always account for all items of income and do not over-claim on expenses.

Retirement

For most people, this is the time of high 'net worth' – your mortgage is hopefully paid off, you may have moved to a smaller home and released capital, insurance policies may have matured and you may have inherited some money along the way. Statistics show that a man retiring at 60 will live for just over a further 21 years and a woman just over 25 years. These days, many doctors are retiring earlier, but early retirement must be planned for.

Recommendations

Take professional advice with regard to pension planning. Currently, there are so many different forms of pension on the market that you will benefit from an independent expert opinion. Your pension should be tailored to your personal circumstances. Also think about passing surplus capital down to your children or their children – this may save taxation in the form of death duties.

Consider the management of your investments. Investment decisions will vary according to the individual – factors will include:

- your age
- your income requirements
- the degree of risk that is acceptable to you

- expectations as to future levels of inflation
- perception of the economic climate.

In general terms, always ensure that where you are in receipt of a pension, your spouse is in receipt of the investment income, against which any personal tax allowances may be allocated.

Do not forget your will – does it need changing? Currently, inheritance tax is charged at a rate of 40% on all estates in excess of £234 000. In retirement, make use of annual exemptions whereby both husband and wife can give away £3000 in any tax year. If the full £3000 is not given in any year, the balance can be carried forward for 1 year only, and is then allowable only if the exemption for the second year is used in full. Where an individual makes an irrevocable gift and survives for 7 years from the date of the gift, no inheritance tax is payable. If the donor does not survive for 7 years, the tax payable is reduced so that only a proportion is charged (Table 14). Always keep a record of gifts for possible scrutiny at a later date.

Table 14

Timing of irrevocable gifts and inheritance tax

Years between gift and death	Tax payable (% of full amount due)
3–4	80
4–5	60
5–6	40
6–7	20

Avoiding the pitfalls

Be wary of passing on to younger generations such amounts of capital that you may compromise your ability to pay for nursing home fees in the future.

Do not worry about spending appropriate amounts of capital in retirement if your pension does not allow you to maintain your standard of living.

Try not to die as the 'the richest person in the graveyard' – inheritance tax, currently at a rate of 40%, means that considerable amounts will have to be paid even after personal relief.

medicolegal matters

Gerard Panting MA MRCGP DMJ
Head of Policy and External Relations,
Medical Protection Society

*"The best place for a lawyer in a hospital is
on the operating table and not sliding
around causing trouble for other people."*
Frank Dobson,
The Royal College of Midwives, 1998

The law governing medical practice has evolved to such an extent that medical law has become a flourishing specialty in its own right. Doctors are subject to multiple systems of accountability. As a consequence, one clinical incident may give rise to a series of investigations, some of which may not be completed for years after the events in question. It is important that you understand clearly your responsibilities from the outset of your career and keep them in mind thereafter. This chapter covers the major issues that may arise during a typical medical career. As in every other area of practice, it is important to know the limits of your own expertise and seek help earlier rather than later if you are in danger of straying beyond them.

Confidentiality

Confidentiality is an important legal as well as ethical principle. The basic rule is that information obtained in professional confidence should be divulged only with the consent of the individual concerned. However, the rule is not absolute and there are some common exceptions.

- Information must be disclosed when there is a statutory duty (i.e. one laid down in legislation), for example, notification of an infectious disease, termination of pregnancy, stillbirth, birth or death.
- If a court order requires you to disclose confidential information, failure to do so may amount to contempt punishable by imprisonment or a fine, or both. Doctors served with a formal court order should comply with it, but the mere threat of being served with a court order is insufficient grounds to justify disclosure of information.
- Disclosure is permissible when required in the public interest.
- Most medical treatment is now provided by teams of doctors rather than individuals. Implied waiver assumes (unless there is a direct statement to the contrary) that the patient would wish team members to share relevant information necessary to further the best interests of the patient without specific consent.

Duty to disclose

There are some instances when a doctor has a positive duty to disclose information. The GMC's guidance on confidentiality states, 'Disclosures may be necessary in the public interest, where a failure to disclose information may expose the patient or others to risk of death or serious harm. In such circumstances, you should disclose information promptly to an appropriate person or authority'.

The guidance goes on to quote three examples. The first, a patient who continues to drive against medical advice when unfit to do so. The second, a colleague, who is also a patient, placing patients at risk as a result of illness or a medical condition and, third, disclosure necessary for the prevention or detection of a serious crime. The appendix to the GMC's booklet on confidentiality sets out detailed guidance on disclosure of information about patients to the Driver and Vehicle Licensing Authority (available from the GMC).

you have a **duty to disclose information** when it is in the **public interest**

Medicolegal matters

Consent to treatment

For consent to treatment to be valid, three conditions must be satisfied.

- The patient must be competent to give consent.
- The patient must have sufficient information to make a choice.
- Consent must be given freely.

In law, it will be assumed that adult patients are competent to consent, but this assumption is rebuttable (i.e. a person challenging you on this point may be able to show that the individual in question was not competent, so you should always assess competency on a patient-by-patient basis).

The competent patient must be able to:

- comprehend the treatment information provided to him, and
- believe it, and
- weigh it in the balance to make an informed decision.

The level of information that should be given to a patient prior to canvassing consent is a common cause of debate. Before making that decision, consider:

- the degree of risk
- the severity of risk
- the risk:benefit ratio of the treatment
- the patient's mental state.

Although it is up to you to decide what information should be given to your patient, this is not a licence for medical paternalism. The GMC has now issued detailed guidance on consent, *Seeking patients' consent: the ethical considerations*, which sets out standards more demanding than current case law. The booklet is available from the GMC and is essential reading for all doctors. Remember that questions must be answered honestly and as fully as the patient demands. If you believe that the patient will suffer serious harm to his mental or physical health through disclosure, withholding information may be justified.

Just because a patient is under the age of 16 years, do not assume that he or she is incompetent. A child who is able to understand the implications of accepting or rejecting a specific treatment is as competent as an adult. In most circumstances, you will probably consider it good practice to seek to persuade the child to inform a parent, but when a competent child adamantly refuses and providing treatment would be in the child's best interests, you should proceed and maintain confidence.

Those deemed not competent

Not all patients are competent to give consent. In the case of minors (those under 18 years of age in England and Wales, and 16 years of age in Scotland), consent to medical, dental or surgical treatment may be obtained from any person with parental responsibility for the patient. However, in the case of adult patients who are incapable of giving a valid consent, no one, not even the court, has the power to give consent by proxy. In these circumstances, treat the patient in accordance with his best interest as would be judged by a responsible body of medical opinion.

Advance directives/living wills

Where a patient is no longer able to give or withhold consent, but has previously – when competent – given a clear instruction about future treatment, that wish should be respected even if it amounts to refusal of treatment that might be life-saving. A classic example would be a Jehovah's Witness admitted to hospital unconscious and bleeding but with a clear written statement refusing blood or blood products in any circumstances. However, problems are likely to arise if:

- the advance directive does not specifically apply to the patient's current condition
- the patient's instructions are vague and open to interpretation
- there is a good reason to believe that the patient has had a change of heart since making the declaration.

If the advance directive does not appear valid or applicable to the patient's current condition, the doctor should treat the patient in accordance with his best interests.

Consent forms

Consent forms are not, in themselves, absolute proof that valid consent was obtained to the treatment specified on the form. Most consent claims are 'failure-to-warn' cases, with the claimant arguing that he would not have consented to the treatment if the full facts had been explained. Whenever you counsel a patient prior to a procedure, discuss the pros and cons of the proposed treatment and available alternatives, and answer the patient's questions fully. It is useful to make a note of the main areas discussed.

Medicolegal reports

Few doctors will complete a medical career without having to prepare a medicolegal report at some stage. Before putting pen to paper, it is essential that all relevant documentary evidence, including the medical records, are to hand.

Your report should start with a brief summary of your personal details, such as:

- your qualifications, with dates gained
- your experience in the specialty prior to the current post
- the date of your appointment to your current post.

Sometimes it is necessary to explain the staffing or other attributes of a particular unit or to give background information about the patient.

A detailed, factual account of your personal involvement in the patient's care should now be set out, written in the first person singular ('I') and devoting a separate paragraph to each contact. In some instances, you will be asked to comment on points made in legal documents or the statements of others. If so, comments must be objective. Use the same numbering system as that used in the original document. If you feel vulnerable to criticism, seek legal advice immediately.

Clinical records

In the NHS, it is the responsibility of the Trust to retain medical records, whereas in private practice responsibility rests with the individual clinician. So how long should medical records be kept? The counsel of perfection is to keep everything forever – however, this is not practical.

Competent adult patients dissatisfied with the outcome of their treatment have 3 years from the date of becoming aware of potential problems to commence proceedings. The vast majority of cases will have declared themselves by 10 years, so this is taken as the minimum retention period for medical records of competent adult patients. Obstetric records should be retained for 25 years and records of paediatric patients should be retained until the patient's 25th birthday or 10 years after the completion of treatment, whichever is the later.

Medical records should be kept securely and, when no longer needed, destroyed by shredding or incineration.

The importance of accurate clinical records cannot be over-emphasized. Complaints, claims of negligence and other forms of investigation may not materialize for weeks, months or even years after the events in question. By this time, you are unlikely to remember exactly what happened at a given consultation, particularly when there was a sequence of consultations over a period of time. Even if only for corroboration, you must be able to refer to contemporaneous medical records – if they are inadequate, your position will be prejudiced.

> inaccurate records may **prejudice** your **position** should **complaints arise**

An adequate medical record is one that enables you to reconstruct the consultation without you having to rely on your memory. It should include:

- details of the history
- answers to relevant direct questions
- a record of all systems examined, noting all positive findings and important negative findings, as well as objective measurements, such as blood pressure and peak flow
- the clinical impression formed
- any investigations ordered
- any treatment prescribed or referral made
- arrangements for follow up.

Medical records should also be objective and worthy of independent scrutiny as, in the event of an investigation, notes will be pored over in considerable detail.

At first, this may seem a daunting task, far too onerous given the time available during the consultation, and an unnecessarily defensive response to the rising tide of negligence claims and complaints. But this is not defensive practice: the primary purpose of a medical record is to provide continuity of care and all the details referred to above are necessary to meet this end. Coincidentally, the notes will be of considerable evidential value. In addition, good medical records will create a good impression of the doctor's general standard, whereas shoddy notes will be equated with shoddy practice. Keeping comprehensive medical records is an intrinsic part of good medical practice – defensible rather than defensive practice.

Responding to complaints

Should something go wrong, the patient and/or relative (subject to confidentiality considerations) is entitled to a full and frank explanation of why things happened in the way that they did. However, before attempting to explain, you should establish the facts. For this, you will be reliant on adequate medical records, the paucity of which may have been the root of the problem in the first place.

Most hospitals deal with complaints via a nominated complaints officer who will coordinate responses from all staff involved. Sometimes, face-to-face meetings may be arranged. The complainant may be angry and appear aggressive. If so, allow him to say what he wants to say without interruption but paying due attention. Then address the points raised in order, allowing him to ask supplementary questions along the way. Be empathetic and do not hold back from expressing sympathy. When something has gone wrong, be prepared to apologize – an early apology prevents more claims than prevarication. Also, be prepared to say what has been done to rectify any system failure identified within the investigation.

Clinical negligence

One of the biggest concerns of medical practitioners today is the threat of legal action on the grounds of negligence. The annual number of medical accidents in the NHS is around 300 000; of these, around 82 000 arise from incidents of medical negligence. In May 2000, the National Audit Office reported that the NHS was faced with bills amounting to £3.4 billion for medical negligence claims. Yet most doctors are surprisingly unaware of the basic requirements for a successful legal action.

Civil negligence

This is the most usual course of action. A successful claimant would be awarded damages. The court will base its decision in such cases 'on the balance of probabilities' (referred to as the burden of proof).

In order to be successful, the claimant must show that (on the balance of probabilities):

- he was owed a duty of care by the doctor/hospital
- the duty was breached
- he suffered harm as a result of that breach of duty.

There is rarely any argument over the existence of the duty of care between the doctor and his patient. It is far more difficult to determine whether or not the care provided reached a reasonable standard and if not, what damage, if any, resulted from the shortfall in care. It is not enough to point to harm suffered by the patient and poor standards – the two must be causally related for compensation to be payable.

The standard of care provided by medical practitioners is judged by reference to the 'Bolam test'. This simply states 'A doctor is not guilty of negligence if acting in accordance with a practice accepted as proper by a responsible group of medical men skilled in that particular art.' In other words, to be defensible, the doctor must be able to call upon experienced colleagues in that specialty who will testify that the doctor's management was reasonable. So, the question is not whether your action was right or wrong, but whether you acted reasonably.

Inexperience is no defence. If you know that a particular procedure, or foreseeable complications arising from that procedure, requires a level of skill or expertise beyond your own, you should refer your patient to a more experienced colleague. Giving it your best shot is simply not good enough.

Similarly, when delegating duties, it is incumbent upon you, as the delegating doctor, to ensure that the person (whether medical or non-medical) to whom the task is delegated possesses the necessary qualifications, skills and experience to carry out the procedure to a reasonable standard.

The development of protocols and guidelines may reflect a consensus view on best management of particular conditions. Failure to follow that guidance may not, in itself, be negligent, but is likely to mean that you now have to justify – by reference to a responsible body of medical opinion – why management was varied in an individual case.

Compensatory awards of damages are designed to restore the patient (in so far as money ever can) to the position they would have been in had negligence not occurred. Damages are divided into general damages for pain, suffering and loss of amenity, and special damages to compensate for loss of earnings and special needs, including such things as adaptations to the home, specially adapted cars, employment of staff and private remedial therapy. Compensation payments are not made on the basis of the seriousness of the mistake but the impact of the negligence on the patient's life. At the time of writing, the record award in the UK in a medical negligence case stands at £4.5 million.

Criminal negligence

Some acts of medical negligence resulting in death are deemed to be so reckless as to warrant criminal prosecution. Unfortunately, there is no clear-cut definition of the degree of negligence that warrants criminal prosecution. The law relies upon the rather circular argument that cases to be prosecuted are those where the doctor's conduct was sufficiently bad to require prosecution. In such a case, the burden of proof is 'beyond reasonable doubt'.

The expert witness

Lord Woolf, now Lord Chief Justice but until recently Master of the Rolls (the most senior judge in the civil courts in England and Wales) was asked to conduct a review of the civil justice system. In his final report, he stated that expert evidence was one of the two major generators of unnecessary cost in civil litigation and stated that the expert's duty is to assist the court impartially on matters within his expertise. Rule 35.3 (Civil Procedure Rules) states:

1. It is the duty of an expert to help the court on matters within his expertise.
2. This duty over-rides any obligation to the person from whom he has received instructions or by whom he is paid.

Expert evidence is given in a written report, unless the court directs otherwise, that must be made available to other parties in the case. They then have 28 days in which to submit (once only) written questions, which must be for the purpose of clarification only, to the expert. Replies to those questions are then treated as part of the expert report. If questions remain unanswered, the court can decide that the party may not rely on the evidence of the expert or that his fees may not be recovered from another party.

At the end of an expert report, there must be a statement by the expert that he understands and has complied with his duty to the court. The body of the report must state the substance of all material instructions, whether written or oral, on which the report has been based. These instructions are not privileged against disclosure.

Lord Woolf was very keen to encourage discussion between experts that might serve to reduce the number of issues in contention. The idea has found favour with most doctors, but some lawyers are reluctant to allow it for fear they may prejudice their case. However, the court may now direct experts to meet to discuss contentious issues.

The court may specify the issues to be discussed and direct that, following their meetings, experts prepare a statement for the court. The statement should detail the issues on which the experts agree and disagree, and include a summary of their reasons.

Experts have the right to file a written request to the court for directions to assist them in carrying out their function – and may do so without giving notice to any of the parties to the action. This provision gives the expert a means of dealing with improper practices or pressures from parties or their legal advisers, and recognizes the new over-riding provision that the expert serves the court above all others.

Availability of experts

The following is an extract from the Times Law Report *Matthews v Tarmac Bricks and Tiles Ltd.*, 1 July 1999, and is self-explanatory.

"Doctors who held themselves out as practising in the medicolegal field had to be prepared so far as was practical to arrange their affairs to meet the commitments of the court."

"It was very important that in cases where doctors were involved as much notice as possible was given for the date of the hearing. However, it was essential that it be appreciated that whereas the courts would take account of the important commitments of medical men, they could not always meet those commitments in a way that would be satisfactory from the doctor's point of view."

"Ways had to be found to meet the obvious requirement that cases should be heard expeditiously. That required cooperation between the parties, members of the medical profession and the courts."

"The message which had to be understood by both the medical profession and the legal profession was that it was essential if parties wanted cases to be fixed for hearing in accordance with the dates which met their convenience, that those dates should be fixed as early as possible."

Coroners' inquests (England, Wales and Northern Ireland)

The purpose of a coroner's inquest is to determine who, when, where and by what means a person died. It is inquisitorial in nature and may be a prelude to civil litigation or further investigation by the GMC or the police.

Any death should be reported to the coroner if:

- no doctor treated the patient in his last illness, or saw the patient within 14 days of death, or after death
- the death occurred during or after surgery
- the death was sudden and unexplained or if there are suspicious circumstances
- the death might be due to an industrial injury or disease, accident, violence, neglect, any kind of poisoning or abortion
- the death occurred while the person was in legal custody or where there are allegations of negligence.

Following a report, the coroner's officer, often a retired police officer, will usually ask all clinicians involved in the patient's care to provide a report (see *Medicolegal reports*, page 125). Should you feel open to criticism, seek independent expert advice from your medical protection society immediately.

You, and indeed any interested party, may be legally represented at an inquest. The normal indications for representation are when:

- you feel vulnerable to criticism
- the coroner has indicated that you may be criticized

- the family is to be legally represented
- there is substantial press interest.

Law evolves, and doctors must keep abreast of developments governing medical practice. Reliable sources of information include the *BMJ*, the journals of the medical protection societies and risk management publications.

In Scotland, the Procurator Fiscal conducts Fatal Accident Inquiries in roughly the same circumstances.

Further reading

Copperfield T. How to take the law into your own hands. *Hospital Doctor* 1996;23 May:41–2.

Department of Health. *Supporting Patients, Protecting Doctors*. London: Department of Health, 2000.

DHSS. *Informed Consent, HC(90)22*. London: HMSO, 1990.

General Medical Council. *Good Medical Practice*. London: GMC, 1998.

General Medical Council. *Seeking Patients' Consent: The Ethical Considerations*. London: GMC, 1999.

General Medical Council. *Confidentiality*. London: GMC, 2000.

General Medical Council. *When Your Professional Performance is Questioned*. London: GMC, 1999.

Hood CA, Hope T, Dove P. Videos, photographs, and patient consent. *BMJ* 1998; 316:1009–11.

McLean S. *EL(97) 32 Consent to Treatment – Law and Ethics in Medicine*. Glasgow: Glasgow University, 1997.

Ward S. Laying down the law on medical evidence. *BMA News Review* 1994;June:21–2.

Warnock M, Doyal L, Tobias JS *et al.* Informed consent in medical research. *BMJ* 1998; 316:1000–5.

Winder E. Prevention and control of clinical negligence. *Clinician in Management* 1994;3(suppl 1):15.

Medicolegal matters

success in medicine: voices of experience

When this book was conceived, a selection of 'the great and the good', as well as some of our special friends and colleagues, were invited to give their own recipe for success in medicine.

Charles A Akle BSc MS FRCS

Independent General Surgeon, Harley Street, London

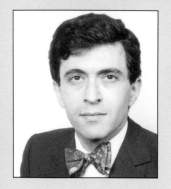

Sir Derek Dunlop used to teach that there are three ingredients for success in medicine: intelligence, good looks and money. At the turn of the century, three different ones were suggested: a top hat for authority, a paunch for dignity and piles for an anxious expression (anonymous, *The Lancet*). More recently, the secrets of success in private practice are considered to be the three As: ability, affability and availability.

The truth is there is no guaranteed formula for success because the definition of success is subjective. For some, it is financial reward, while for others it is achieving one's vocation and serving one's fellow man. Some might consider a contribution to modern science or recognition by one's peers or society to be a measure of success.

In my personal experience, there are several factors that contribute to success: hard work, a willingness to learn and adapt to new information, a desire to improve continually the quality of one's work by self-analysis and peer review, an ability to communicate well and, above all, good manners. Add to these a large dose of luck. Of all these, perhaps the ability to communicate well is the key as it is important to all of the other factors, particularly when combined with the rarest of commodities, insight. Nearly always, those who fail have no insight into their behaviour or lack of communication. Nevertheless, it is incredible how certain doctors who are appalling diagnosticians, poor communicators and poor practitioners of their art can achieve success, be it in academic or clinical work. There is hope for everyone!

Of course, if you do have pots of money, astounding good looks and a modicum of intelligence, you may well enjoy what you consider to be success. But when you are dead and gone, nobody will regret your passing. I wonder if it really matters?

Success in medicine

Peter Amoroso MB BS FRCA

Consultant Anaesthetist, Deputy Regional Advisor, Training Programme Director,
Barts and the London School of Anaesthesia

Teaching is fundamental to the role of a doctor. Our ability to teach is a measure of our success. We can all recall our favourite teachers who, by their enthusiasm and clarity of thought, imparted knowledge that has remained with us throughout our careers. These mentors enjoy a special form of success that makes them the most accomplished of all doctors. Today, there are numerous courses available for the would-be teacher. At consultant interview, all short-listed candidates have the requisite clinical and academic skills, but few demonstrate a genuine commitment to teaching and education. These abilities can win the day.

The GMC has clear guidelines for the doctor as a teacher. The teacher should be a role model by acting as a clinical and educational supervisor to junior colleagues. *Professional* attributes highlighted are a consistently high standard of professional and personal values relative to patients and their care, and ensuring one's availability or accessibility to patients. Effective communication skills, demonstrable personal professional development and a commitment to team-working are prerequisite. *Personal* attributes include an enthusiasm for one's specialty, together with an understanding of the processes of assessment and appraisal of the trainee. The Royal Colleges, the Deaneries and the Specialist Training Authority support the training needs and competence of staff in this capacity.

Teaching methods have changed considerably in recent years. The formal environment of the lecture theatre has given way to more interactive methods, such as tutorials, seminars and problem-based learning, which encourage trainee participation. The techniques for oral presentations, writing papers and abstracts together with computer skills help us to teach more effectively. With the advent of revalidation, clinical governance and continuing educational and professional development, good medical practice will require us all to be competent, effective and enthusiastic teachers.

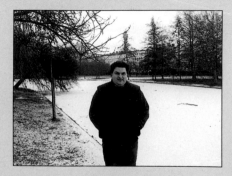

Dame Josephine Barnes DBE DM FRCP FRCS FRCOG FKC

Consulting Gynaecologist, Charing Cross Hospital and Elizabeth Garrett Anderson
Hospital, London and Past President of the British Medical Association

There are various points that are worth considering in the ambition to succeed in medicine.

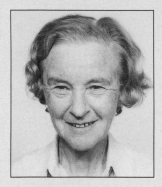

- You will have chosen your medical school and will be admitted. You may of course be a mature student with a previous degree, or someone starting from scratch. It doesn't really matter; both do equally well.

- Realize that some years of really hard work, not very well rewarded, lie ahead of you; you must be prepared to accept this. You will have to attempt – and pass – a number of examinations, so it is important to develop your examination technique. As an examiner, I would say that the most important thing is to write your papers, if you have to, very clearly so they are easy to read. Think of the poor examiner, reading the paper at 3 o'clock in the morning!

- Aim to marry the right person and stay married. This is always helpful. Your partner may be medical or from a paramedical background, and this again may prove to be helpful, provided there is no conflict of interest.

I was inspired by our Professor of Obstetrics, FJ Browne, an outstanding teacher and an equally charming man. I think it is due to him entirely that I decided that obstetrics and gynaecology was the right thing for me.

I have had the advantage of serving for some time on the Council of the Medical Defence Union. I also have two brothers who are lawyers, so I have a fair view of the pitfalls of medical practice, including actions for negligence, which indeed are becoming more and more common. If you are threatened with legal action, do not despair. Good help is available, and it is important that you consult your defence society immediately. Do not sit back and think that it will go away, because it may not. You may have to give evidence in court, and the most likely, in your junior days, is in a coroner's court. Remember to address the bench – that is the coroner, not the barrister who is questioning you. Give your answers clearly in simple language as they will be written down. In some cases, you may be submitted to fairly tough examination or cross-examination. Relax. Take it in your stride. The barrister is only doing his job.

Avoid the obvious pitfalls of drugs, drink and adultery. Remember that the most important way of achieving success in medical practice is to have a good reputation.

Dame Josephine Barnes provided this contribution shortly before she died on 28 December 1999, aged 87.

Professor Michael Daum ChM FRCS

Chairman of the Council of the National Institute of Medical Humanities and Professor of Surgery, Royal Free and University College Medical School, London

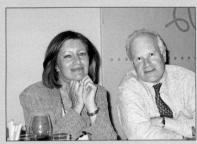

I was flattered to be invited to contribute to *Succeeding as a Hospital Doctor*. This suggests that some folk judge me to have been a success; paradoxically, my career has been plagued by my sense of inadequacy and a need to prove myself constantly. Even today, with three Chairs and a Higher Merit Award tucked under my belt, I still feel that I am only as good as my last operation or publication (perhaps, then, this is the secret of success – never give in to a sense of complacency).

My career, as I look back at it now, falls into two distinct segments: my period of training up to my achieving the status of Senior Lecturer, and my career as an academic surgeon.

My early and relatively rapid progression through the ranks can, I think, be attributed to an almost pathological degree of conscientiousness. I worked long and hard, not so much to curry favour with my mentors, but out of an intense sense of responsibility for all my patients. I view with despair the current attitudes among junior surgical staff who expect to achieve the same level of expertise with shorter hours and shorter training programmes.

The success I have enjoyed as an academic surgeon has, I believe, been built on my parallel interest in art, literature, philosophy and the humanities. My love of literature and the theatre has helped me to develop programmes for improving communication skills and the psychosocial support of my patients. My readings around the history and philosophy of science have taught me to question the 'received wisdom'. The teachings of Karl Popper encourage my lifetime dedication to proper scientific method, of which the randomized, controlled trial in the evaluation of treatments for breast cancer is a classic example. In my past few years as a clinical academic, I am spending more and more time developing a curriculum and teaching my undergraduates about the importance of the humanities in the development of a successful medical career.

The final secret of my 'success' is to have chosen my wife wisely. Without a stable and happy home life, success in medicine is an illusion.

When I followed my father and grandfather into the family practice in 1962, I was referred to as 'the young Dr Bogle'. Not being prepared to spend my career with this label, I decided that I must create my own identity within the medical profession.

Earlier in 1962, while working as a pre-registration house officer, I looked after an 8-year-old girl – Sally – who was in terminal renal failure. I spent many hours talking to her and counselling her parents. I was devastated when she died, but had learned much about dispensing care, sympathy and compassion.

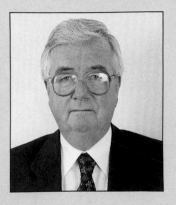

Working in Liverpool presented me with the opportunity to represent residents in their opposition to the local authority's draconian rehousing policy. For the first time in my life, I found that I had the ability to lead people in fighting injustice, to be articulate in presenting their case, and to succeed in changing views. This led me to take up the challenge of Sir James Cameron (a former Chairman of the BMA Council) who, when I asked him what he was going to do to improve my life as a GP, replied that I should help myself by working through the Local Medical Committee and the BMA. This was the most significant conversation in my professional life.

Keith Bush MB BS MD(Lond)

Consultant Orthopaedic Physician, Past Honorary Consultant Orthopaedic Surgeon,
The Royal National Orthopaedic Hospital Trust, London

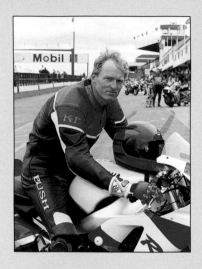

Succeeding means different things. In my case, it is an endless supply of interesting patients with intellectually challenging problems that I generally have a practical solution to. It is also important to have gained the respect of ones' peers and to be invited to teach.

The most important factors in achieving this success are the desire and the luck, and appropriately directed hard work to take advantage of this. Reasonable intelligence, mental and physical health, and energy are blessings. My mother sacrificed a great deal to give me a good education. I injured my back while at medical school, which was frustrating at the time, but ultimately lucky. It opened my eyes to the fact that back pain was not well understood and gave me the desire to learn more. I was lucky to learn from James Cyriax, a pioneer in the field of musculoskeletal medicine.

Doing clinical research over almost 20 years while in full-time clinical practice was very, very time-consuming. However, the experience gained in one's chosen field and the resultant doctorate are invaluable.

Make time to listen to your patients and find out what their problem means to them. Make time to think, to perfect techniques and to network.

Success in medicine

It is, if anything, a combination of good luck and good judgement that has given me what I now have. Whether it is 'success' is for others to decide.

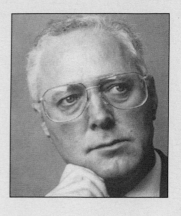

I chose, when bedridden, frustrated and bored, to read a large book about the electrocardiogram. As I worked my way through the book, I became keen on the subject and expert at interpreting the traces. From that time on, I was hooked. Although I tried to do something 'better' – surgery, for instance – I was always pulled back to medicine and cardiology because of an unusual expertise in this particular investigation.

When well into the throes of cardiology, I noticed that the most exciting topic was cardiac electrophysiology. It had just started and was obviously a subject that had far to go, and would go far. I got involved in it quickly, found the most experienced clinicians and the best scientists, and adopted them as role models. It was not too difficult; the work was long and hard, but there was little competition. It took little more than a year or two to be close to the top in terms of skill and experience. Everything was new and needed to be written up. Although not a natural writer, I linked up with friends who were. We wrote voraciously, published much and then turned to higher degrees.

Then I had to make some decisions. Should I stick to an ultra-specialty? Should I work in a teaching hospital? Would it be more sensible to take an academic job? From my perspective, 'yes' was the answer to all of these questions; the combination of a professorial job, in a highly specialized area, seemed right. After that decision, all went according to plan.

The recipe was:

- identify a new and important subject
- develop the necessary expertise
- work with role models and with friends
- recognize what you can do well and what you do badly
- take opportunities, but not risks.

Succeeding as a hospital doctor

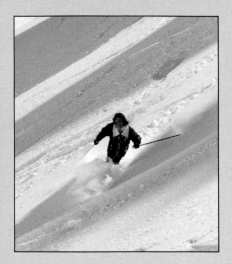

Success in medicine – as in any other career – can be judged in many different ways and I am not sure that I would consider myself to be successful. Some think of me as intolerant and undiplomatic with a dreadful bedside manner. I don't really like hospitals or the way in which the NHS is currently being managed, nor do I approve of the new system of training doctors. In addition, I can't cope with ill health in myself, family or friends; so I am not really the ideal doctor. However, I am enthusiastically dedicated to my career in medicine and have developed my own ten commandments.

1. You really can have your cake and eat it. Don't believe anyone who says you cannot have a successful career in clinical medicine with a good reputation in your hospital, an international research profile, a busy private practice and a happy family life – it is possible, you just have to engineer it. Work hard, play hard – it is not worth doing the former without the latter.

2. Appropriate time management is essential. Don't waste time. I was influenced by Golda Meir's autobiography *My Life* in which she emphasized the importance of striving to do a little more each day than she had managed during the previous one. Punctuality at work is essential, not only does it set a good example and stop the trainees from turning up late, but it ensures that the operating lists don't overrun, thus pleasing the anaesthetist and theatre staff. However, social activities can often be delayed and no one really minds or even notices when you go round to a friend's half an hour or even an hour late, giving you time to get your slides ready for tomorrow's lecture or mark the last few exam papers before you go.

3. Delegate – it is not possible to do everything yourself, nor is it desirable. The people you train usually do things your way, only better, so let them.
4. Think to whom it matters most. Whenever you have a dispute at work or at home, try to be one who gives in unless you are absolutely certain that winning is essential to you. It is not worth upsetting people for something that is of minor importance.
5. Don't 'criticize' your colleagues. You never know when you'll need their help. Try to support them when they are in dispute with others and don't be frightened to ask for their help when you need it. Protect your boss – everyone is hungry for something and you are bound to need him for a reference, surgical training or teaching in the future.
6. Develop a way of saying 'no' without causing offence. It is flattering to be asked and tempting to accept all invitations to lecture, operate abroad, examine and write, but it is impossible to do it all. Try to judge which events it would be possible to miss and offer a member of your team instead.
7. Give others the opportunity to do things they wouldn't have otherwise been able to do. This applies to patients, colleagues, family and friends. Don't do it for them, but give them the facilities, advice, time and financial aid to do it for themselves. It is much more rewarding for you and for them.
8. Make use of all the support services you can. It is much quicker to earn the money to pay a secretary to do the typing, a cleaner to do the housework and a gardener to mow the lawn than it is to do it yourself. If at all possible, marry an understanding spouse and teach your family to appreciate that medicine isn't just a job, it's a way of life.
9. It's not enough to fulfil your contract, you have to show commitment by starting early, staying late and taking on extra tasks, including teaching, research and committee work.
10. Enjoy life – if you are not happy most of the time, then change tack. Life is too short to spend time being miserable!

Professor Ian Craft FRCS FRCOG

London Gynaecology and Fertility Centre Limited, London

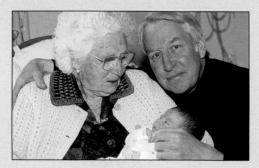

Professor Craft with his mother and IVF godchild

Application, commitment and dedication to the acquisition of knowledge and skills are the hallmarks of success in medicine. Nothing is as enlightening as repeated exposure to clinical situations. Resolute commitment, tenacity in adverse circumstances and attention to detail have certainly assisted me in my career, leading me to become a specialist in one sphere of medicine. I also have a strong ethos about being a team player.

However, my career has not been one of flawless success. I was a sensitive child and failed my 11 plus. Insecurity in exam situations continued with poor O level results (two passes out of seven), but insecurity gave way to confidence when, at the age of 15, I met my future wife, then aged 13. I have not failed an exam since.

My early interest was in farming but I decided not to pursue this as my family had limited financial resources and I would have had to be a tenant farmer, thus preventing me from controlling my own destiny – something that is important to me. My decision to pursue medicine came rather like the conversion of Paul and stemmed from being enthused after reading George Sava's *The Healing Knife*. The book portrays a caring and compassionate doctor and, after making a personal commitment to do something similar, I have never strayed from my course. In addition, there is a strong aspect of determination in my character.

I chose to specialize in obstetrics and gynaecology, with my competitive nature leading me to aim for a teaching hospital position. However, this was not to be – my inherent interest in research, with almost 50 papers published by the time I was a senior registrar, practically predetermined an academic career. I have always been fascinated by creation, hence my later involvement in reproductive medicine. Being very much a team player, I set up the *in vitro* fertilization programme at the Royal Free Hospital that was to result in the birth of Britain's first test-tube twins (1982). My former wife says that I'm not afraid of anything, and perhaps my willingness to 'walk on thin ice' is the reason I have been successful – I do not see the problems that deter others from pursuing a similar course. Without my wife's support, I do not believe that I would have been so creative or successful. We remain the closest of friends and have the utmost respect for each other, having been through so much together.

I was taught by some excellent teachers at both the Westminster Hospital and the Hammersmith, and also at Queen Charlotte's where I became a senior lecturer prior to being appointed to the Chair of Obstetrics and Gynaecology at the Royal Free Hospital. After 6 years here, I became concerned about the restrictions of undertaking an academic career on limited research funding and decided, together with the core of my team, to run an assisted-conception clinic in the independent sector, while still pursuing as much clinical research as possible. We are now located at the London Gynaecology and Fertility Centre. I also established an assisted-conception programme in Dubai, with the Department of Health and Medical Services of Dubai, which provided services not in existence previously.

I am certainly not afraid of controversy and am prepared to be radical if I believe the cause to be in the patient's best interest, and tend to be passionate about many issues, medical and otherwise. I believe life is for living to the full and one needs a counterbalance of outside interests in order to cope with the stresses of a demanding medical career. In my circumstances, this involves a passionate interest and commitment to the arts, as well as a fascination with nature and heritage. I am happiest when out walking alone or with a companion in wild places, carrying my binoculars.

It has been a privilege for me to work in medicine as I feel my team and I have made a contribution in our own small way. Despite radical changes in the structure of the National Health Service since I entered it, I still believe that medicine is a fulfilling career if one is totally committed to its practice. It certainly has been for me.

Finally, I would like to recall the philosophy behind George Sava's book. Despite wonderful advances in medicine, to be caring, compassionate and able to offer kind words are attributes we should all strive to attain.

It helps to succeed in medicine if you remember that it is not only a science, but an art too. I interned in the USA, alongside colleagues better technically trained than me. However, they placed much less emphasis on communication with patients than me. I quickly saw how important it is to not only be able, but also be willing to communicate with patients – in terms of improved patient compliance, avoiding confrontations with patients or relatives, fostering a more realistic attitude to what medicine can and cannot do – for example, being able to tell a patient that there is nothing more that can be done while still maintaining a fruitful doctor–patient relationship.

Many doctors, indeed most of us, work in situations in which being able to accept the limits of what they can do is absolutely essential to their survival as doctors. A number of very wise physicians have taught me that medicine's therapeutic enthusiasm, essential for the most part, has its own drawbacks. Doctors can have difficulty accepting their limits, and end up making such needless and pointless effort.

Finally, there is the issue of pacing yourself. Read William Osler's *A Way of Life* and ponder his regret that many a young medical life has been

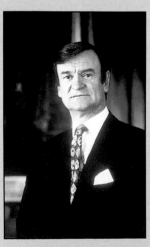

wrecked by too fast a starting pace, a hustle, bustle and tension, 'the human machine driven day and night'. Avoid what William James has called 'those absurd feelings of hurry and having no time', and always leave room for the important things in your own personal life – your loves, family and friends. That way you can, even in the most awesomely demanding situations, call each day your own and be not just a good doctor but perhaps even a great one.

Professor Liam Donaldson MSc MD FRCS (Ed) FRCP FRCP (Ed) FFPHM

Chief Medical Officer, Department of Health, London

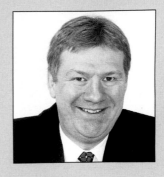

"Medicine is a noble profession." So replied a prospective applicant to medical school whom I interviewed years ago when asked why he wanted to be a doctor. Throughout my career in medicine, I haven't seen too much evidence of nobility, but I have found that an undue obsession with status or too great a fondness for the trappings of high professional life can be dangerous traits. A doctor who is an autocratic leader, who regularly has disputes with colleagues or who is unable to see the world through the eyes of the ordinary patient is likely to be associated with dysfunctional clinical teams, risking poor outcomes for patients.

After training in surgery, I moved into epidemiology and public health, initially in an academic role and later as director of public health for one of the NHS regions. For 6 years, I combined this role with that of regional director (effectively chief executive). Appointment as the Government's Chief Medical Officer means that I have now worked in all six sectors that make up British healthcare – hospital medicine, primary care, public health, academic medicine, management and the Government service.

I have learned that while the technical tasks of medicine are important, it is at the level of the team, the service and the organization that good healthcare is generated. Achieving results through people and managing change is a universally difficult task and one that few are skilled in, trained or prepared for. Many of tomorrow's doctors will be in leadership roles. They will need to create the culture in which excellence in clinical decision-making can flourish.

Many of the qualities needed are well captured in the expression 'the reflective practitioner'. Someone who is willing to learn and change, someone who is willing to listen, someone who seeks feedback on their performance and someone who is willing to reassess a misunderstanding is more likely to take the right decision in a complex clinical situation or when the future of a service is being debated. Such a person is more likely, too, to gain the respect of peers and colleagues as a clinical leader.

Succeeding as a hospital docto

Professor John Fitzpatrick MCh FRSCI FRCS

Professor of Surgery, University College Dublin, Ireland and
President of the British Association of Urological Surgeons

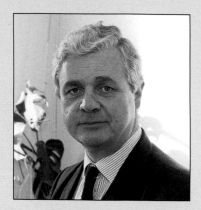

A successful career depends on a combination of several factors. First, be good at networking. Always be friendly when first introduced to someone. Be sensitive to the wishes of those you meet and take the time to find out what matters to them. Avoid making enemies as they may harbour a grudge for many years.

Recognize opportunities as they arise. If you allow opportunities to pass you by, you may never achieve your full potential. As your career develops, it is important to be decisive. Process paperwork efficiently rather than allowing it to pile up. Aim to arrive at meetings early and sometimes, if appropriate, leave before the end; few important decisions are made towards the end of a meeting when people have already begun to leave.

Finally, never agree to chair meetings unless you intend to do it properly; if you do not, you risk being associated with failure. Chairing a meeting is a challenge, but enables you to create an aura of success and convey your point of view more easily than as a member of a committee. As chairman, allow everybody to have their say, but stop participants speaking for longer than their allotted time. Give preference to those who raise their hand to speak rather than those who interrupt; in this way, you can maintain control of the discussion.

These are only a few of my thoughts on success. As in Desert Island Discs, if I had to decide which factor was the most valuable or desirable, it would be that one should strive to be open and friendly, as well as expert and honest in communication with everyone at all times.

Professor Brian G Gazzard MA MD FRCP

Consultant Physician, Chelsea & Westminster Hospital, London

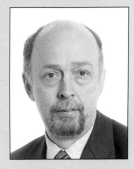

Surely the true measure of success is 'Are you eager to go back to work each day, do you feel fulfilled and is the pay cheque an unexpected and largely irrelevant bonus?' By this yardstick, there are many unsung heroes in our profession and there are many academics who have failed.

I started life as a gastroenterologist. In 1979, I encountered my first AIDS patient and my life changed irrevocably. Confronted by young patients destined to die, I had to learn to watch the process and 'be there' for them. It was their courage and acceptance that allowed my staff and me to carry on. We were also privileged to be able to do what doctors have been trained to do ever since Sir William Osler's day:

- to observe acutely
- to describe new algorithms of care
- to find new treatments.

Medicine has recently come full circle and many individuals will now survive this horrific disease if we can convince them to take the treatment.

The secret of success in medicine, as in life, must be time management – spend at least part of each day doing something that is worthwhile for you. Also, at the end of each day, spend a brief period evaluating what has happened and renewing your vows not to continue to do what you hated doing that day.

Medicine remains an art. We have swung too far with Higher Education Funding Council annual reviews of achievement towards a narrow concept of peer-review publications and hard grant money as the criteria of worth. The question of whether patients feel better as a result of seeing you – albeit a much more difficult concept to quantify – is an infinitely more valuable indicator of your own success. Knowledge, lateral thinking, communication skills (particularly the talent of listening) and, the most basic of all, a sixth sense that all is not well with your patient. All these contribute to your success. They are, of course, difficult to teach – learn them from your peers as an apprentice would learn from a master. They will make all the difference to your success as a doctor.

Succeeding as a hospital doctor

Just about everything I have done outside the surgery has stemmed from the Edinburgh fringe. The five summers that I spent there were not only the most enjoyable of my life, but also gave me the opportunity to learn most of the skills that I now use for lecturing and broadcasting. We (the double act Struck Off and Die) were very fortunate to corner an area of the market – black medical humour – that no one else was attempting in public. Thanks to some shocking reviews and seven reports to the Broadcasting Standards Council, our notoriety spread.

Although we tried to fight the case of junior doctors, it soon became apparent that satire doesn't change anything – nobody takes comedians seriously. So, in 1991, I approached Ian Hislop in the toilets at a BBC Radio Light Entertainment Christmas party and asked him if he'd like a medical column in *Private Eye*. A month later and *Doing the Rounds* was born. I started exposing the plight of junior doctors but my mailbag was soon full of all sorts of NHS scandals, including the 'Bristol cardiac disaster'. I wrote about it four times in 1992, specifically bringing it to the attention of the

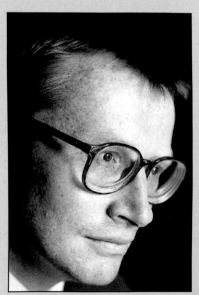

Health Secretary and the relevant professional bodies. I eventually realized that no one takes *Private Eye* seriously either.

I was offered *Trust Me, I'm a Doctor* partly because of my 'warts and all' attitude to medicine, but also because none of the other doctors auditioned was prepared to criticize his profession in public. At last, a chance to be taken seriously. Well, sort of. The audience is relatively small (around 2 million) and nothing of the 24 episodes has ever been reviewed in the medical press. There is still – quite understandably – an antipathy towards media medics and, despite my smug exterior, I don't particularly enjoy exposing just what a patchy service the NHS provides. But, if you go into the mainstream media, you're forced to see everything from a patient's perspective rather than a doctor's. If your child was having heart surgery, would you like to know how many operations the team has done, what their results are and how they compare with the national average?

To survive in the media, you have to be thick-skinned, self-obsessed and competitive. You have to be able to cope with bad reviews and a steady trickle of hate mail. And if you're married with kids, you have to keep things in perspective. So it's a lot like medicine. But with one crucial difference. A medical position is still as close as you can get to having a job for life, whereas Dr Ginger-Smug could be axed from your screen at any time. My work is, currently, varied but, as the critic Victor Lewis Smith wrote of the first series of *Trust Me, I'm a Doctor*, "The words 'day job, up the' and 'don't give' spring to mind."

Bill Hendry MD ChM FRCS

Consultant Urologist, St Bartholomew's and Royal Marsden Hospitals, London and
Past President of the British Association of Urological Surgeons

I believe the most important single attribute that leads to success, whether in medicine or in other fields, is enthusiasm. Fortunately, enthusiasm is not something that you are born with: it can be acquired. Like a fire, enthusiasm must be sparked initially. Thereafter, it should be fuelled; finally, it can be fanned into flames that cannot be extinguished.

Just so in medicine, a great teacher shares enthusiasm for his subject

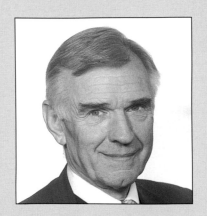

with his students. Whether it be cardiac surgery or cataracts, volvulus or varicose veins, the intense interest of the individual teacher is conveyed. In my case, it was kidney disease that first stirred enthusiasm: young people dying of uraemia while a dialysis machine lay in the next room, only used for acute reversible renal failure. The idea of organ transplantation was not new, but the dream of new organs to replace those that had failed inspired an enormous international effort that saw kidney transplantation become a reality.

Enthusiasm is catching. A teacher with a needle-sharp mind, absolute clarity of vision and communication skills can shed light where before there were obscurity and darkness. We have all seen the results – a group of students fired into activity, competing to produce the best dissertation, and falling over each other to get onto the ward round or into the operating theatre, questions waiting to be answered. And life choices to be made: will it be medicine for the thoughtful, surgery for the practical or pathology for the reflective? So long as there is enthusiasm, success is sure to follow.

Why have I had a successful career? Who knows? Certainly not me, having never been party to the reasons why, against strong competition, I have been appointed to various positions of responsibility. Chance certainly played a part – being in the right place at the right time – but clearly there is more to it than that. I believe commitment, diplomacy and a dedication to obeying the Golden Rule have contributed to my success.

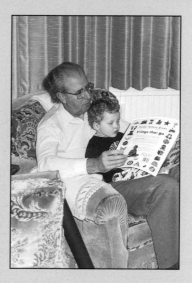

Commitment enabled me to pass exams with high marks in the early years, and has kept me up to date as the years have progressed. Diplomacy enabled me to avoid making enemies while never being a wimp; it also helped others take notice of my point of view. And the Golden Rule – do unto others as you would have done to yourself – has guided me in clinical practice at all times. Happiness and good fortune in my family life has also been of great importance.

My advice to those setting out on a career in medicine is to always admit to and learn from your mistakes. They will become fewer as time passes, but nobody, however senior, is immune.

Michael James Kellett MA MB BChir FRCR

Consultant Radiologist, University College London Hospitals and Honorary
Senior Lecturer, Institute of Urology and Nephrology, University College London

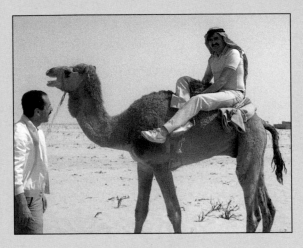

Recently, there have been several documentaries on the life of the junior doctor. I found the negative bias of these depressing as in no interview did the houseman or registrar state that they enjoyed their work. Perhaps I have been lucky. I chose to enter diagnostic radiology as I was intrigued by the visual aspect and the diagnostic challenge. As a Dutch colleague later said, "It's rather nice to be paid to look at pretty pictures." I wonder how many of us, 30 years ago, would have foreseen the dramatic and clinically relevant changes that were to take place in radiology.

The student X-ray tutorials at Bart's were under the strict guidance of the Bart's/Brompton radiologist George Simon. He would grill us mercilessly on 'the chest X-ray'. I learned the first lesson in student survival, which was to pass through the pain threshold of such a critical tutorial and emerge holding the tutor in the highest respect, and we certainly respected George.

As a junior radiologist, I was impressed by the strong team approach of Ian Kelsey Fry, Bill Cattell and John Wickham to the clinical problems at the weekly clinico-radiological conference at Bart's, and this was to lead me towards a career in uroradiology.

Early in my radiology training, it became clear that this was a specialty that was likely to expand more than any other although I did not expect such colossal changes as we have seen. This expansion has been in two directions: the explosion of cross-sectional imaging (I was with Ian Kelsey Fry when he set up the first private CT scanner in London) and the technical advances in interventional radiology.

When looking for a consultant post in radiology, I would pass on the advice given to me by Ian Kelsey Fry, which was to give more time to assessing and networking with your clinical colleagues than your radiological colleagues, for it is through the clinical contact that patient referrals and hence job satisfaction occurs. On my appointment to St Peter's Hospital, I had the advantage of working closely with the most famous names in British urology. I soon became interested in interventional radiology as I saw the huge benefits of simple needle and catheter manipulations to patients. Central to this was the enthusiastic encouragement I received from the inspirational John Wickham, who really was the first to have the concept of a team approach to minimally invasive therapy.

Sir Alexander Macara DSc FRCP FRCP (Ed) FRCGP FFPHM DPH FMedSci HUM

Chairman of the Council, British Medical Association 1993–98

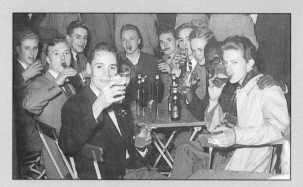

Tivoli Gardens, Copenhagen 1954. Sir Alexander (front left) accompanying a group of medical students to Denmark

When I took up my first post as Lecturer in Public Health in 1963, I was naturally expected to inspire students with a passion for statistics, epidemiology, the organization of healthcare and the relevance of the social sciences to medicine. I realized that I was doomed to failure unless I could demonstrate the relevance of the social aspects of medicine. I did this by constructing a 4-week course in which the students studied how people live and work, and how they are helped or hindered by their environment and the people who serve them, not only in healthcare. My approach drew deep scorn from many senior colleagues, including the Professor of Medicine. When I was working with him on an epidemic of hepatitis, he taunted me over lunch to justify what use it would be to doctors to have visited slums and gone down mines. Realizing that he was not joking and that I had to provide an answer, I hit upon the revolutionary idea of making an objective evaluation of the students' response to my course. There was no medical model to be found for this, but my educational sources identified a formidable lady, Ruth Bowden, who had developed a model of evaluation in her own field. It had the essential qualities of simplicity and objectivity, requiring students to assess every element of the course in terms of value (as perceived by them at that stage in their studies), interest and presentation.

The students responded with delight that they were being consulted for the first time and, to the discomfiture of conservative colleagues in the faculty, insisted upon surveying, with my help, the whole curriculum. The outcome was not only more teaching time for social medicine, but the opportunity to involve over 200 general practitioners throughout the region in demonstrating the essential contribution of primary care to the curriculum.

There was an unexpected bonus. My professor and mentor, Robert Wofinden, one of the last great Medical Officers of Health, was invited to contribute to the first meeting of a World Health Organization-inspired Association of Schools of Public Health in Europe (ASPHER). In the customary way, he invited me to write a paper for him in which I reviewed the outcome of this work. Sadly, at short notice he was unable to attend the meeting, and I went to Zagreb in his place, delivered my own paper on his behalf and consequently became Secretary General of ASPHER shortly afterwards. Thus was I launched upon the international career that has so greatly enriched my life's work.

Professor Alan G Johnson MChir FRCS

Professor of Surgery, University Surgical Unit,
Royal Hallamshire Hospital, Sheffield

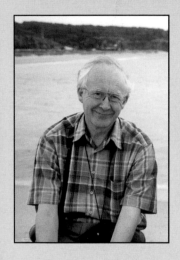

What is success? The answer to that question depends on which criteria are used, and who is making the judgement – the patient, the employer, the audit office, the bank manager, colleagues or God. It is easy to confuse the apparent trappings of success – income, size of car, appointments and honours – with the real thing: that is, the quality of service to patients and the profession. I collect quotations and aphorisms, many of which have been constant companions throughout my career. 'People matter more than things' and 'The patient is the centre of the medical universe, about which everything else revolves' (Lister) have helped keep the right perspective when commitment to patients has been threatened by bureaucracy, petty regulations, trivia or quick gains. It is tempting to try to manipulate your own affairs (and other people's) to gain a top position, only to find that you have to stay there by the same techniques. It is important to do apparently mundane jobs well, without a continual eye on the quick chance for self-promotion, because reliability and integrity are enduring qualities that gain credibility and respect in the long run.

However, success can have its cost – cost to family, health, personality or values. Some of the worst advice I have read is 'knife before wife', suggesting that family relationships should be sacrificed for single-minded surgical success. Some years ago, I was very pleased at being invited to be a guest speaker at three international conferences, one after the other. However, I was taken ill and had to cancel all three visits. As I was lying in bed, frustrated at missing such an opportunity, my daughter came home from school, sat on my bed and commented, "Daddy, we like it when you are ill – we can get to know you." It only needs a few words to put academic achievement in perspective. After all, it was Jesus Christ who warned, "What good would it be for a man if he gains the whole world, yet forfeits his own soul?"

Success in medicine

Professor J Gordon McVie MD FRCP

Director General, The Cancer Research Campaign

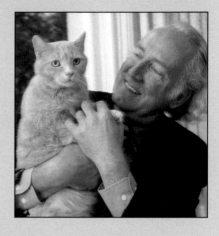

I suppose to end up in a job as a Director General of a cancer charity might well not be seen as succeeding in medicine, rather it would be seen as failing! However, I suppose I became a consultant at 31 because I was in a novel specialty and I was around at the right time. Anti-cancer drugs were just being developed in the early 1970s. I was in an excellent clinical pharmacology and haematology unit and was lucky enough to be given training in the USA, thanks to the late Gordon Hamilton-Fairley, the first Professor of Medical Oncology in the UK. He was blown up, tragically, as most people will remember, by mistake by an IRA bomb. So how did I get to the consultant job at an early age? An outstanding professor, who gave me a rope long enough to hang myself, and a determination, particularly after Hamilton-Fairley's death, to pick up the reins and fill the gap – I think if you ask any number of medical oncologists why they are doing what they are doing, they will also attribute the motivation to Hamilton-Fairley. But more fundamentally, I had started off life with genetically endowed curiosity. This was hammered out of me at school while I swotted for exams to escape from school and I hum-drummed my way through university only finding the library when invited to do an honours degree in pathology! There I recovered my curiosity within the library and it has not been dampened since!

I have found the following proverbs and epigrams particularly apt with regard to my own career, remembering the most useful definition of a 'career' is that it is the name given to all those crazy decisions one has made in the past 20 years.

- Montgomery said, "There is only one rule in war – never invade Russia". Always identify and avoid impossible tasks.
- Having decided that you are going to have a crack at something, remember the motto of the Chindits – the boldest course is the safest.

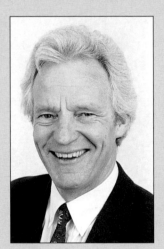

- Success in a project is often the result of chance, failure the result of bad planning and execution; failures are more important than successes for learning.
- Never put your faith in organizations, only in people.
- Fortunate is the doctor whose main source of stress is his patients; most doctors I know have more stress caused by colleagues.
- It is easier to seek forgiveness than permission.

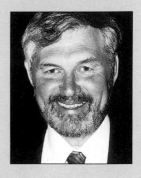

I believe that in every field of human endeavour, a key factor in success is not to be afraid of change. The practice of medicine and structures of service delivery have changed dramatically throughout my career and will no doubt continue to do so.

I trained in an era when the patient expected the doctor to be the fount of all knowledge – quite a daunting prospect for the inexperienced house officer or young general practitioner. However, I quickly learned not to encourage this dangerous myth. Never be afraid to be open with patients and admit that you don't have all the answers.

This is particularly relevant in the light of the recent explosion in information technology. Medical information and in particular 'cutting edge' research, previously only available to the profession, can now be accessed by anyone on the Internet. Increasingly, patients arrive at consultations clutching reams of print-outs detailing symptoms and treatments for conditions they have or believe that they have! In this context, our role as doctors is to assess the information and advise the patient on its relevance to them.

This leads on to another important principle, that of involving patients in decisions regarding treatment. If patients feel that they have played a meaningful part in the decision-making process, they are more likely to take your advice and comply with any treatment prescribed. It is essential that patients in the terminal stage of life should play a major part in setting the agenda for whatever time remains to them. The doctor's task is to help the patient and family make the treatment choices that will deliver the best possible quality of life throughout whatever time is left. In this respect, we have a great deal to learn from the hospice movement and I always advise young people contemplating a career in medicine to try to spend some time working in a hospice before making their decision.

Despite the long hours and heavy responsibilities, medicine remains a fascinating and rewarding occupation. If I had my life to live again, I would still, without hesitation, choose to be a doctor.

Succeeding as a hospital doctor

Professor Eric J Thomas MD MRCOG FMedSci FRSA

Dean, Faculty of Medicine, Health and Biological Sciences,
University of Southampton and Vice Chancellor (Elect), University of Bristol

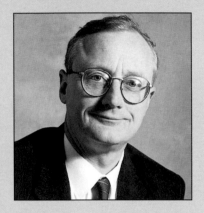

We are immensely privileged to belong to a profession that addresses problems of major relevance to the population, presents us with considerable intellectual and moral challenges, and is both well respected in society and very secure. The privilege has to be earned and recognition of that fact should be the mainstay around which our careers are built.

More practically, there are four factors that I consider to be crucial to success.

- Be a good clinician – it is the bedrock of your career.
- Plan your career – think about what you want to be. Freud defined life as "to love and to work", thus placing work at the very emotional centre of existence. However, I remain astonished by the number of senior trainees who have not completed the dialogue with themselves and their families about what they wish to achieve, where and why. It's very hard to get to a place if you don't know where you're going.
- Work very hard and fulfil your deadlines (e.g. acquire special clinical skills, write the MD, publish that difficult paper). Doctors who think that they are the only individuals who have to work hard in order to achieve success are naïve – look at trainees in commerce or law.
- Finally, constantly place medicine within broader political and social dimensions – this ensures a sense of perspective and a realization that we are embedded in society, not separate from it. This will serve your career well generally, but particularly in the most senior positions, where successful interaction with government, the civil service and higher education is necessary.

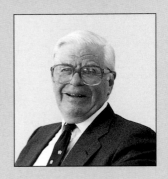

I can only excuse my immodesty in contributing to this book by reminding myself, and you, that what a young surgeon needs for success, beyond a modicum of native wit and some manual dexterity, is luck. Luck in finding agreeable and influential mentors. Luck in being in the right place at the right time and gaining that vital appointment. Luck with one's patients. And luck in acquiring good assistants and dependable staff in wards and theatres.

Everyone needs to be a specialist in something. During my residency at St Peter's Hospital, London, a child was admitted with congenital urethral obstruction. I soon perceived that the St Peters' staff knew nothing about children, while the Great Ormond Street expertise in paediatrics did not stretch to urology. Thus I spotted a gap – and in a very exciting field at that. Although adult surgery was more remunerative, paediatric surgery became my area of expertise. It afforded me the opportunity to publish on issues unfamiliar to most urologists.

Older surgeons need the chance to move on to a different field before their incapacity to master the newest techniques becomes too painfully obvious. Happily for me, I assumed the Directorship of the British Postgraduate Medical Federation. Although the position involved some difficult and vexatious challenges, it broadened my horizons considerably and led on to some fascinating experiences working with many of our professional bodies.

Professor Dame Margaret Turner Warwick DBE DM
(Oxon) PhD (London) FRCP

Emeritus Professor of Medicine, University of London and Past President of the Royal College of Physicians (London)

The following are my personal principles in medicine and in life in general.

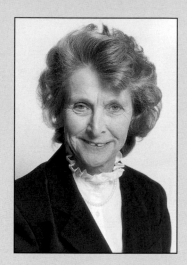

- In clinical medicine, I believe in a blend of optimism and realism, and, above all, sharing this with patients.
- Ignore gender. It is irrelevant to medicine.
- Take professional opportunities as they arise; over-planning rarely works. For example, as a registrar in the 1950s, I undertook the impossible task of the hospital autopsies when the pathology service was in temporary abeyance. This not only restored the teaching service within the hospital and my learning, but formed the basis of a PhD thesis!
- In medicine, the real reward is the unrepentant fulfilment of giving professional support and help to individuals in need, but this is dependent on seeing the job through. Patients want continuity of care; it forms the basis of experience on which quality medicine depends. Reconciling this with modern patterns of 'care' is one of the main challenges in the NHS. The solution probably depends on the difference between closely coordinated teams of seniors, juniors and other healthcare professionals – mutually respecting each other's special expertise, *but working together* – and not the many much looser, less satisfactory shift-work systems.
- We all have our limitations. Thus a truly seamless service of primary, secondary and tertiary care is the only way to run an economic, efficient, quality NHS. Easy referral of patients to someone who may know more should be regarded as a personal strength, not a weakness. There is no place for territorial complacency in medicine.

- The amount we *do not* understand fully in medicine vastly exceeds that which we *do* know. The current emphasis on 'guidelines and protocols' – modern variants of general statements on medical practice, previously summarized in multi-edition, fully referenced textbooks! – forms an essential basis for medical management. However, guidelines must always be recognized as such, and balanced against a doctor's judgement, given the individual and their particular circumstances.
- Leading a professorial department should, in my view, be likened to the approach of Atlas; the opposite of top-down. You should support and promote both clinical and research opportunities to enable others to develop – and bask in their glory as they go from strength to strength.
- Medicine is a remarkable field and is probably uniquely rewarding. No other profession combines one-to-one relationships with patients, an opportunity to contribute to national standards of medical practice through a variety of managerial involvement, teaching and learning from home and overseas undergraduate and graduate students, clinical research that covers real bedside-to-bench medicine and the persuit of one's own special interests in dialogue with other international experts – *all at the same time*.
- Having an endlessly supportive husband, children and grandchildren is strongly recommended.

The several definitions of 'success' in the Concise Oxford Dictionary include "the attainment of wealth, fame, or position". Medically, this might encompass strings of degrees, a Harley Street address, a university professorship, high office in the establishment, titles and, to crown it all, a lengthy obituary in *The Times* (ideally appearing in error before one's demise).

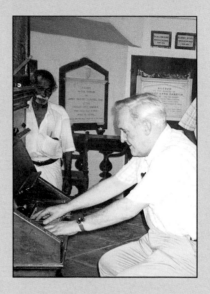

But can these accolades be equated with genuine success? Or do they just happen to some individuals by dint of hard work, ability or driving ambition, and, above all, good luck? Certainly, they do not come to equally deserving people or necessarily bring with them the satisfaction of being your own man or woman. They do not provide a sense of being at ease with yourself, or the genuine fulfilment of having done at least one thing to the very best of your ability, or even just a little better.

Is it ever possible to achieve these infinitely more worthwhile facets of success? Mentors are useful, if for nothing else, as living evidence of mistakes not to be made. Here are a few. First, do not plan your life or career in obsessive detail; those who do rarely achieve self-fulfilment or happiness. Take plenty of time to learn the basic clinical and communication skills or, if you have the burning curiosity necessary to follow a research career, the essential tools of the trade. Have a long look, both at home and abroad, at the many faces of our wonderful profession before deciding in which direction to proceed, and who to travel with. To achieve the satisfaction of doing at least one thing really well, focus on something really absorbing in a continuously self-critical way, but try to retain a broad view across medicine and the humanities. Ignore those who say there is only one pathway to career development; take some risks and be your own person from the beginning.

Remember that, although medicine is a noble profession, there is no intrinsic difference between an effective doctor and an able high-court judge or thorough roadsweeper. That occupational hazard, pomposity, is a danger to patients and precludes any possibility of coming to terms with yourself, warts and all. Pace your life and learn to say 'no'; a mind refreshed by something other than medicine or turgid administration is much more effective in the clinic or research laboratory. Later, treat young people with respect and understanding, however stupid and impossible they may seem; with increasing age, the pleasure that you will gain from their success will go some way to balancing your inevitable failures. Finally, find a partner who is sympathetic to the many trials and few successes of what, if you follow this advice, will not always be an easy ride.

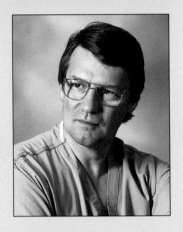

Surgery is a very practical subject that must be led from the front by those with technical expertise. Cardiac surgery is more an obsession than a career. I decided to be a cardiac surgeon at the age of seven, when the first open-heart operations by Lillehei and Kirklin featured prominently in the media. I never wanted to be a 'proper doctor' and made my ambitions clear at the medical school interview. I was captain of cricket and rugby, and without taking a prize exam, my single-mindedness was recognized with the award 'Student Most Likely to Succeed'. In 1972, I won a scholarship to the USA and spent the time in a cardiac surgical unit in New York and a trauma room in Harlem.

Subsequently, I was made house physician and house surgeon to both academic units at the Charing Cross Hospital. After the primary FRCS, I was appointed to my first cardiac surgical post as resident surgical officer at the Brompton Hospital.

During my general surgical training in Cambridge, I was nicknamed 'Jaws' and operated on anything and everything day and night, and by the time I returned to cardiac surgery as registrar at the Hammersmith Hospital, I had an enormous hands-on general surgical experience. The heart is unforgiving and should never be the first target organ for a trainee surgeon. Soon afterwards, I took a research fellowship with John Kirklin at the University of Alabama (1981). This was the most stimulating environment in cardiac surgery of that era, and my research on complement activation and the post-perfusion syndrome provided a thesis and career-long research interest.

Britain's lead in cardiac surgery began to dwindle rapidly, as private practice took surgeons out of NHS hospitals. At this time, I visited the USA and learnt the technical skills that consolidated my affinity for the US approach.

In 1986, at the age of 37, I was appointed consultant to the new Regional Cardiothoracic Unit in Oxford. This presented the unique opportunity for a new direction in cardiac surgery as there were no senior colleagues. A cardiac recovery area was established within the operating suite, and a so-called 'fast-track recovery' model was pioneered. Within a few years, the number of operations increased from 150 to 1800 patients per year and the 'fast-track' model was adopted worldwide for straightforward cases.

A new challenge arose in 1994 when I met the artificial heart engineer Robert Jarvik and began a collaborative programme with the Texas Heart Institute to pioneer the new miniature Jarvik 2000 artificial heart.

I believe the foundations of my early career – a huge volume of surgery, continuous innovation and a flare for presentation whether written, spoken or in the form of international surgical workshops and demonstrations – were of tremendous value. The Grim Reaper sits on the shoulders of every cardiac surgeon, but the more competent the technician, the higher becomes his surgical mortality through selective case referral. This requires certain self-defence mechanisms including good health, both physical and mental, unerring confidence in one's own ability, and a stable and supportive family life.

useful addresses

Action Research
Vincent House
Horsham
West Sussex RH12 2DP
Tel: 01403 210406
Fax: 01403 210541
Email: info@actionresearch.co.uk
www.actionresearch.co.uk

Arthritis Research Campaign
Copeman House, St Mary's Court
St Mary's Gate, Chesterfield
Derbyshire S41 7TD
Tel: 01246 558033
Fax: 01246 558007
Email: info@arc.org.uk
www.arc.org.uk

Association of Medical
Research Charities
29–35 Farringdon Road
London EC1M 3JF
Tel: 020 7242 2472
Fax: 020 7242 2484
Email: info@amrc.org.uk
www. amrc.org.uk

Association for the Study of
Medical Education (ASME)
4th Floor, Hobart House
80/82 Hanover Street
Edinburgh EH2 1EL
Tel: 0131 225 9111
Fax: 0131 225 9444
Email: info@asme.org.uk
www.asme.org.uk

Biotechnology and Biological
Sciences Research Council
Polaris House
North Star Avenue
Swindon
Wilts SN2 1UH
Tel: 01793 413200
Fax: 01793 413201
www.bbsrc.ac.uk

British Medical Association
BMA House
Tavistock Square
London WC1H 9JP
Tel: 020 7387 4499
Fax: 020 7383 6400
Email: smanley@bma.org.uk
www.bma.org.uk

BMA Counselling Services
(BMA members only)
Tel: 0645 200169

Brain Research Trust
Bloomsbury House
74–77 Great Russell Street
London WC1B 3DA
Tel: 020 7636 3440
Fax: 020 7636 3445
Email: thebrt@aol.com

Breakthrough Breast Cancer
6th Floor, Kingsway House
103 Kingsway
London WC2B 6QX
Tel: 020 7430 2086
Fax: 020 7831 3873
Email: info@breakthrough.org.uk
www.breakthrough.org.uk/docs

British Heart Foundation
14 Fitzhardinge Street
London W1H 4DH
Tel: 020 7935 0185
Fax: 020 7486 5820
www.bhf.org.uk

British Postgraduate
Medical Federation
33 Millman Street
London WC1N 3EJ
Tel: 020 7831 6222
Fax: 020 7831 7599

Cancer Research Campaign
10 Cambridge Terrace
London NW1 4JL
Tel: 020 7224 1333
Fax: 020 7487 4310
Email: crcinformation@crc.org.uk
www.crc.org.uk

Department of Health
Public Enquiry Office
Richmond House
79 Whitehall
London SW1A 2NL
Tel: 020 7210 4850
Email: dhmail@doh.gsi.gov.uk
www.doh.gov.uk

Engineering and Physical Sciences
Research Council
Email: infoline@epsrc.ac.uk
www.epsrc.ac.uk

European Commission
200 rue de la Loi/Wetsraat 200
B-1049 Brussels, Belgium
Tel: 0032 2299 11 11
www.europa.eu.int

Faculty of Dental Surgery
The Royal College of Surgeons
of England
35/43 Lincoln's Inn Fields
London WC2A 3PN
Tel: 020 7312 6667
Fax: 020 7973 2183

Faculty of Occupational Medicine
6 St Andrew's Place
Regent's Park
London NW1 4LB
Tel: 020 7317 5890
Fax: 020 7317 5899

Faculty of Public Health Medicine
4 St Andrew's Place
Regent's Park
London NW1 4LB
Tel: 020 7935 0243
Fax: 020 7224 6973
Email: enquiries@fphm.org.uk
www.fphm.org.uk

Fellowship of Postgraduate Medicine
12 Chandos Street
London W1M 9DE
Tel: 020 7636 6334
Fax: 020 7436 2535

General Medical Council
178 Great Portland Street
London W1N 6AE
Tel: 020 7580 7642
Fax: 020 7915 3641
Email: gmc@gmc-uk.org
www.gmc-uk.org

**Higher Education Funding Council
for England (HEFCE)**
Northavon House
Coldharbour Lane
Bristol BS16 1QD
Tel: 0117 931 7317
Fax: 0117 931 7203
Email: hefce@hefce.ac.uk
www.hefce.ac.uk

Imperial Cancer Research Fund
61 Lincoln's Inn Fields
London WC2A 3PX
Tel: 020 7242 0200
www.icrf.org.uk

Institute of Healthcare Management
7–10 Chandos Street
London W1M 9DE
Tel: 020 7460 7654
Fax: 020 7460 7655
Email: mailbox@ihm.org.uk
www.ihm.org.uk

**Joint Centre for Education
in Medicine**
33 Millman Street
London WC1N 3EJ
Tel: 020 7692 3145
Fax: 020 7692 3109
Email: jcentre@tpmde.ac.uk
let.open.ac.uk/jcm/aboutus.htm

**Joint Committee on Higher
Medical Training**
c/o Royal College of Physicians
5 St Andrew's Place
Regent's Park
London NW1 4LE
Tel: 020 7935 1174
www.rcp-london.co.uk/jchmt

Joint Committee on Postgraduate
Training for General Practice
14 Princes Gate
Hyde Park
London SW7 1PU
Tel: 020 7581 3232

Joint Committee on Higher
Psychiatric Training
c/o Royal College of Psychiatrists
17 Belgrave Square
London SW1X 8PG
Tel: 020 7235 2351

Joint Committee on Higher
Surgical Training
c/o Royal Colleges of Surgeons
35–43 Lincoln's Inn Fields
London WC2A 3PN
Tel: 020 7405 3474

King's Fund
11–13 Cavendish Square
London W1M 0AN
Tel: 020 7307 2400
Fax: 020 7307 2801
www.kingsfund.org.uk

Macmillan Cancer Relief
Anchor House
15/19 Britten Street
London SW3 3TZ
Tel: 020 7351 7811
Fax: 020 7376 8098

Medical Defence Union
3 Devonshire Place
London W1N 2EA
Tel: 020 7486 6181
Fax: 020 7935 5503
www.the-mdu.com

Medical Interview Teaching
Association (MITA)
Annie Cushing, Honorary Secretary
Department of Human Science
and Medical Ethics
St. Bartholomew's and Royal London
School of Medicine and Dentistry
Turner Street, London E1 2AD
Tel: 020 7601 7522
Fax: 020 7377 7167
Email: a.m.cushing@mds.qmw.ac.uk

Medical Protection Society
33 Cavendish Square
London W1M 0PS
Tel: 020 7399 1300
Fax: 020 7399 1301
Email: info@mps.org.uk
www.mps.org.uk

Medical Research Council
(includes National Institute
for Medical Research)
20 Park Crescent
London W1N 4AL
Tel: 020 7636 5422
Fax: 020 7436 6179
www.mrc.ac.uk

Mental Health Foundation
37 Mortimer Street
London W1N 8JU
Tel: 020 7580 0145
Fax: 020 7631 3868
Email: mhf@mhf.org.uk
www.mentalhealth.org.uk

Migraine Trust
45 Great Ormond Street
London WC1N 3HZ
Tel: 020 7831 4818
www.migrainetrust.org

Muscular Dystrophy Group of Great
Britain and Northern Ireland
7–11 Prescott Place
London SW4 6BS
Tel: 020 7720 8055
Fax: 020 7498 0670
Email: info@muscular-dystrophy.org
www.muscular-dystrophy.org.uk

Multiple Sclerosis Society of Great
Britain and Northern Ireland
25 Effie Road
Fulham, London SW6 1EE
Tel: 020 7610 7171
Fax: 020 7736 9861
www.mssociety.org.uk

National Advice Centre for
Postgraduate Medical Education
British Council
Medlock Street
Manchester M15 4AA
Tel: 0161 957 7218

National Institute for
Clinical Excellence
90 Long Acre
Covent Garden
London WC2E 9RZ
Tel: 020 7849 3444
Fax: 020 7849 3127
Email: ncca@ncca.org.uk
www.nice.org.uk

National Kidney Research Fund
Kings Chambers
Priestgate
Peterborough PE1 1FG
Tel: 01733 704650
www.nkrf.org.uk

National Osteoporosis Society
PO Box 10
Radstock
Bath BA3 3YB
Tel: 01761 471771
Fax: 01761 471104
Email: info@nos.org.uk
www.nos.org.uk

NHS Confederation
26 Chapter Street
London SW1P 4ND
Tel: 020 7233 7388
Fax: 020 7233 7390
www.nhsconfed.net

Overseas Doctors Association
in the UK Ltd
28/32 Princess Street
Manchester M1 4LB
Tel: 0161 236 5594
Fax: 0161 228 3659

Research into Ageing
Baird House
15–17 St Cross Street
London EC1N 8UN
Tel: 020 7404 6878
Fax: 020 7404 6816
www.ageing.org

Royal College of Anaesthetists
48/49 Russell Square
London WC1B 4JY
Tel: 020 7813 1900
Fax: 020 7813 1876
www.rcoa.ac.uk

Royal College of General
Practitioners
14 Princes Gate
Hyde Park
London SW7 1PU
Tel: 020 7581 3232
Fax: 020 7225 3047
www.rcgp.org.uk

Royal College of Obstetricians
and Gynaecologists
27 Sussex Place
Regent's Park
London NW1 4RG
Tel: 020 7772 6220
Fax: 020 7723 0575
Email: coll.sec@rcog.org.uk
www.rcog.org.uk

Royal College of Ophthalmologists
17 Cornwall Terrace
London NW1 4QW
Tel: 020 7935 0702
Fax: 020 7935 9838

Royal College of Paediatrics and
Child Health
50 Hallam Street
London W1N 6DC
Tel: 020 7307 5600
Fax: 020 7307 5601
Email: enquiries@rcpch.ac.uk

Royal College of Pathologists
2 Carlton House Terrace
London SW1Y 5AF
Tel: 020 7930 5861
Fax: 020 7321 0523
Email: info@rcpath.org
www.rcpath.org

Royal College of Physicians
of Edinburgh
9 Queen Street
Edinburgh EH2 1JQ
Tel: 0131 225 7324
Fax: 0131 220 3939
www.rcpe.ac.uk

Royal College of Physicians
of London
11 St Andrew's Place
Regent's Park
London NW1 4LE
Tel: 020 7935 1174
Fax: 020 7487 5218
www.rcplondon.ac.uk

Royal College of Physicians
and Surgeons of Glasgow
232–242 St Vincent Street
Glasgow G2 5RJ
Tel: 0141 221 6072
Fax: 0141 221 1804
www.rcpsglasg.ac.uk

Royal College of Psychiatrists
17 Belgrave Square
London SW1X 8PG
Tel: 020 7235 2351
Fax: 020 7245 1231
www.rcpsych.ac.uk

Royal College of Radiologists
38 Portland Place
London W1N 4JQ
Tel: 020 7636 4432
Fax: 020 7323 3100
Email: enquiries@rcr.ac.uk
www.rcr.ac.uk/enquiries

Royal College of Surgeons
of Edinburgh
Nicolson Street
Edinburgh EH8 9DW
Tel: 0131 556 6206
Fax: 0131 557 6406
Email: information@rcsed.ac.uk
www.rcsed.ac.uk

Royal College of Surgeons
of England
35–43 Lincoln's Inn Fields
London WC2A 3PN
Tel: 020 7405 3474
Fax: 020 7973 2135
www.rcseng.ac.uk

Royal Medical Society
Student Centre
5/5 Bristo Square
Edinburgh EH8 9AL
Tel: 0131 650 2672

Royal Society of Health
RSH House
38A St George's Drive
London SW1V 4BH
Tel: 020 7630 0121
Fax: 020 7976 6847

Royal Society of Medicine
1 Wimpole Street
London W1M 8AE
Tel: 020 7290 2900
Fax: 020 7290 2909
www.roysocmed.ac.uk

Smith and Nephew Foundation
2 Temple Place
London WC2R 3BP
Tel: 020 7836 7922
Fax: 020 7632 0202

Specialist Registration Office
The General Medical Council
178–202 Great Portland Street
London W1N 6JE
Tel: 020 7580 7642

Specialist Register Helpline
Tel: 020 7915 3638

Specialist Training Authority
of the Medical Royal Colleges
1 Wimpole Street
London W1M 8AE
Tel: 020 7495 1928
Fax: 020 7495 0763
www.sta-mrc.org.uk

Wellbeing
27 Sussex Place
Regent's Park
London NW1 4SP
Tel: 020 7262 5337
Fax: 020 7724 7725

Wellcome Trust
The Wellcome Building
183 Euston Road, London NW1 2BE
Tel: 020 7611 8888
Fax: 020 7611 8545
Email: reception@wellcome.ac.uk
www.wellcome.ac.uk